Molecular Pathology of Alzheimer's Disease

Colloquium
Digital Library of Life Sciences

This e-book is an original work commissioned for the *Colloquium Digital Library of Life Sciences*, a curated collection of time-saving pedagogical resources for researchers and students who want to quickly get up to speed in a new area of life science/biomedical research. Each e-book available in Colloquium is an in-depth overview of a fast-moving or fundamental area of research, authored by a prominent contributor to the field. We call these resources 'Lectures' because authors are asked to provide an authoritative, state-of-the-art overview of their area of expertise, in a manner that is accessible to a broad, diverse audience of scientists (similar to a plenary or keynote lecture at a symposium/meeting/colloquium). Readers are invited to keep current with advances in various disciplines, gain insight into fields other than their own, and refresh their understanding of core concepts in cell & molecular biology.

For the full list of available Lectures, please visit:
www.morganclaypool.com/page/lifesci

All lectures available as PDF. Access to the Collection is free for readers at institutions that license Colloquium.

Please e-mail info@morganclaypool.com for more information.

Colloquium Series on Neurobiology of Alzheimer's Disease

Editors

George Perry
Universiy of Texas, San Antonio

Rudy J. Castellani
University of Maryland School of Medicine

This e-book series on Alzheimer's Disease will provide an up-to-date, comprehensive overview of Alzheimer's Disease and dementia from a multidisciplinary perspective, with a focus on disease pathogenesis and translational neurobiology. The major pathogenic proteins will be described and discussed in depth from the perspective of molecular and cell biology, experimental and transgenic modeling, and in-situ phenotypic expression in humans. Added to this will be in depth discussions of all the major pathogenic theories, including the amyloid and tau protein cascades, oxidative stress, involvement of heavy metals, interplay of the endocrine system, issues surrounded cell cycle activation and protein signaling, and important comorbidities that influence human disease such as vascular neurobiology and synucleinopathy. Treatment paradigms and trials as a function of known components of disease pathogenesis will also be described and discussed in requisite detail that reflects the state of the art. As such, the eBook series will provide a "one stop shop" for the aspiring neuroscientist or physician scientist, and will prove an adaptable framework that can be updated going forward, as dictated by new discoveries and the accumulating scientific literature.

Published titles

(for future titles please see the website, www.morganclaypool.com/page/lifesci)

Molecular Pathology of Alzheimer's Disease
Rudy J. Castellani and George Perry
www.morganclaypool.com

ISBN: 9781615046386 paperback
ISBN: 9781615046393 ebook
DOI: 10.4199/C00095ED1V01Y201310ALZ001

A Publication in the
COLLOQUIUM SERIES ON NEUROBIOLOGY OF ALZHEIMER'S DISEASE

Lecture #1
Series Editor: George Perry, University of Texas, San Antonio, and Rudy J. Castellani, University of Maryland School of Medicine

Series ISSN Pending
ISSN [pending] print
ISSN [pending] electronic

Molecular Pathology of Alzheimer's Disease

Rudy J. Castellani
University of Maryland, School of Medicine

George Perry
University of Texas, San Antonio

COLLOQUIUM SERIES ON NEUROBIOLOGY OF ALZHEIMER'S DISEASE #1

MORGAN & CLAYPOOL LIFE SCIENCES

ABSTRACT

Alzheimer's Disease is characterized pathologically by two principal hallmark lesions, the senile plaque and the neurofibrillary tangle. Since the identification of each over 100 years ago, the major protein components have been elucidated. This has led in turn to the elaboration of metabolic cascades involving amyloid-β production in the case of the senile plaque, and phosphorylated-tau protein in the case of the neurofibrillary tangle. The pathogenesis and histogenesis of each have been the source of extensive investigation and some controversy in recent years, as both cascades have been implicated in the pathogenesis of Alzheimer's Disease, relied upon in the diagnostic criteria for Alzheimer's Disease at autopsy, and targeted for therapeutic intervention. With the accumulation of data and expansion of knowledge of the molecular biology of Alzheimer's Disease, it appears that the enthusiasm for successful intervention has been premature. In this book, we detail the discovery and characterization of the major pathological lesions, their associated molecular biology, their relationship to clinical disease, and potential fundamental errors in understanding that may be leading scientific investigators in unintended directions.

KEYWORDS

Alzheimer's Disease, senile dementia, neurofibrillary tangle, senile plaque, amyloid, amyloid-β, tau protein, phosphorylated tau, β-secretase, γ-secretase, presenilin, oligomer, synapse

Contents

CHAPTER 1

Introduction

It is not by accident that the observations of Alois Alzheimer found their way into the annals of science. They marked rather accurately the senile plaques and neurofibrillary tangles now recognized as hallmark lesions, in the condition now referred to as Alzheimer's Disease (AD) [1] (Figure 1.1).

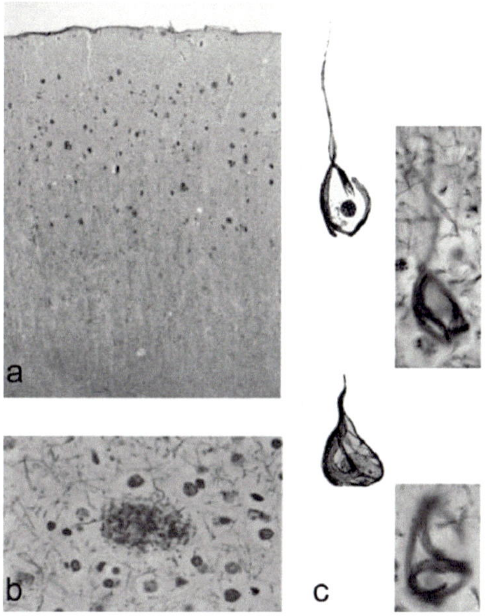

FIGURE 1.1: Tissue sections from Auguste D.'s brain show amyloid plaques (a, b) and neurofibrillary tangles (c) in the cerebral cortex (Bielschowsky silver impregnation). The drawings depicted in c were taken from Alzheimer's own work (1911). Used with permission, the figures were reproduced in Graeber and Mehraein, *Eur Arch Psychiatry Clin Neurosci* 1999; 249 Suppl 3:10–3 [199].

> In sections prepared with the Bielschowsky silver method, remarkable changes in the neurofibrils appeared. In the interior of a cell that otherwise appeared normal, one or several fibrils stood out due to their extraordinary thickness and impregnability. At a later stage, many fibrils appeared, situated side by side and altered in the same way. Then they merged into dense bundles and gradually reached the surface of the cell. Finally, the nucleus and the cell disintegrated, and only a dense bundle of fibrils indicated the site where a ganglion cell had been.

> Since the fibrils could be stained with different dyes than normal, a chemical alteration of the fibrillar substance must have taken place. This then could be the reason why the fibrils survived the death of the cell . . .numerous ganglion cells, particularly in the upper cell layers, had disappeared entirely...[2]

Alzheimer's efforts were emblematic of the productivity of an era in science and medicine that was just beginning to enjoy the benefits of clinical-histologic correlations. Moreover, Alzheimer as an individual was the rare combination of a genuine and humble intellectual, a physician–scientist, and a man of means [3]. Like many seminal observations that led to abrupt advances in the foundation of understanding, both the observations themselves and the individual who made them were equally remarkable (Figure 1.2 and 1.3).

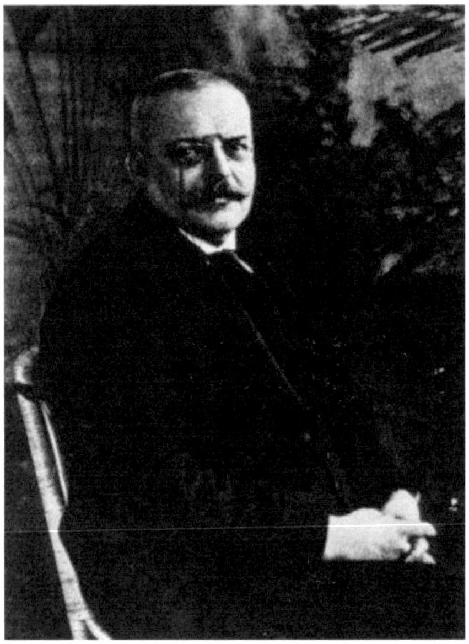

FIGURE 1.2: Alois Alzheimer (1864–1915) was born in the small Bavarian town of Marktbreit, Germany. He received his medical degree from Würzburg University in 1886 and practiced neurology and psychiatry at the Hospital for the Mentally Ill and Epileptics in Frankfurt-am-Main, as well as the Royal Psychiatric Clinic in Munich, among others institutions. Alzheimer is credited with establishing a pathologic substrate for dementia using the Bielschowsky silver impregnation technique. His first two cases were remarkable not so much for the presence of lesions, but for the early age at onset, focal signs, and severity of the pathology. These features were unusual enough to be separated from "dementia senilis," prompting Emil Kraepelin to introduce the term "Alzheimer's Disease," in the 8th edition of his textbook of psychiatry, published in 1910.

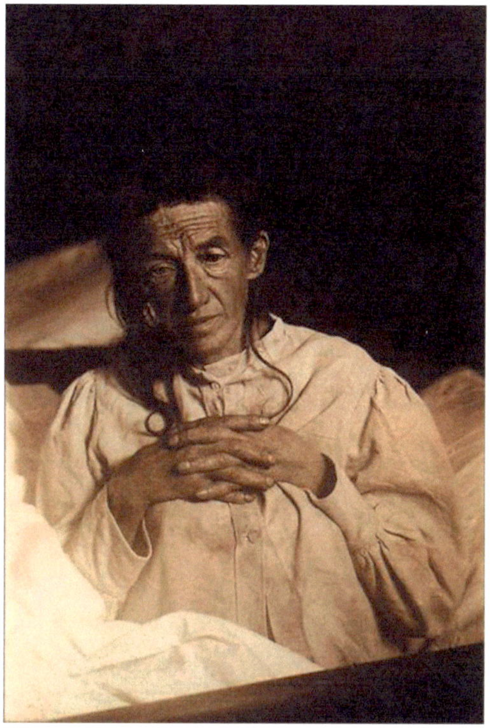

FIGURE 1.3: Auguste Deter was the wife of a railway worker who began suffering cognitive decline in her 40s, eventually presenting for admission to the Hospital for the Mentally Ill and Epileptics, in Frankfurt, Germany, where she was first examined by Alzheimer on November 25th, 1901. She died in April of 1906.

Alzheimer was unusually objective and circumspect about his own data, and he drew conclusions only with care and a measure of doubt. Such is exemplified in the description of his second patient in 1911:

> *"All things considered, we are obviously concerned with a peculiar disease process. Such processes have been established in great numbers in recent years. This finding will necessarily induce us not to be content with laboriously forcing any clinically uncertain case into one of our well-known nosological categories. Doubtless there are many more mental disorders than are listed in our textbooks; in some of these cases histological analysis will allow the peculiarity of the case to be identified later. Then we will gradually reach the point where we will separate single cases clinically from the large nosological groups of our textbooks and define these large groups clinically in a more precise way ..."* [4]

In essence, thorough characterization is necessary to properly define nosological groups, before reaching further conclusions about unusual cases. This kind of genuine objectivity, while seemingly a necessary quality of any scientist in his field, is systemically virtually precluded now more than 100 years later. In a modern era where science has to be sold to funding agencies in order for careers to be maintained if not advanced, where adherence to schools of thought is nakedly prejudicial, and where fealty to senior scientists has less to do with scholarship and innovation than political stratagem, it is somewhat refreshing to peruse the translated works. Moreover, Alzheimer was anything but a self-promoter, as the name of the disease that now bears his name was not put forth by Alzheimer, but his contemporary and boss at the University of Munich, Emil Kraepelin [5] (Figure 1.4). Alzheimer, for his part, went to great lengths to include the observations of others in his descriptions:

> *"Perusini felt that these cases represented a separate disease, partly for clinical and partly for histological reasons. The clinical differences were the early onset, and the presence and severity of focal symptoms, which were not thought to be a feature of* dementia senilis, *the anatomical differences being the greater severity of the histological changes although they develop at an earlier age. Kraepelin still considers that the position of these cases is unclear. Even if the anatomical findings might suggest severe mental impairment, the early onset (one would have to assume a* senium praecox*), the profound language disturbance, spasticity and seizures are very different from those of presbyophrenia, which is usually associated with purely cortical senile changes. The disease may therefore be related to one or to the other of the pre-senile conditions that he described. Fischer has written an exhaustive discussion of Perusini's cases in his paper; 'The presbyophrenic dementia, its anatomical basis and clinical differentiation'. He considered the patches as characteristic of a specific disorder and saw no objections to including in the same category cases occurring at an early age, both because of the histological changes and because the paralysis of adults and young people which represent the disease at a different age share all the essential features of later cases.*
>
> *It seems to me that a simple inclusion of these cases with presbyophrenia does not take sufficient account of several interesting features, and that Perusini's and Kraepelin's reservations against this integration have not been convincingly eliminated by Fischer's arguments. After all, we are dealing with the case of a 56-year-old woman and of Perusini's 46-year-old man, in whom nobody would have made a clinical diagnosis of senile dementia…."* [4, 6]

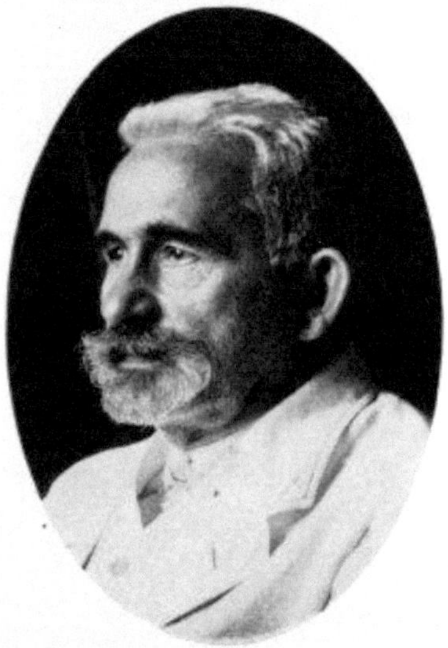

FIGURE 1.4: Emil Kraeplin (1856–1926) was Professor and Director of the Royal Psychiatric Clinic, University of Munich, who recruited Alzheimer to study there in the early 1900s. In addition to numerous contributions to pyshiatry and neurology, Kraepelin was the first to use the term "Alzheimer's Disease" as a form of presenile dementia, as noted above.

Alzheimer practiced both neurology and psychiatry, but with any eye for anatomical observations. He was diligent almost to the point of neurosis in his thirst for the biological basis for human disease. He was at the forefront of neurohistology, his original observations being made possible by employing the Bielschowsky silver technique which was developed only a few years before Auguste D. came to autopsy [7] (Figure 1.5). He thus combined both neuropsychiatric observation and the most basic and cutting edge of human biology, which was the tendency of only a small cadre of exceptional investigators at that time.

Still, a third quality was necessary for this fortuitous combination of talent and technology to come together and push discernibly forward the frontiers of biomedical science. In 1894, Alzheimer married Cecilia Geisenheimer, an independently wealthy widow of a diamond dealer [3], whose fortune supported Alzheimer's research and permitted him to pursue his scientific interests according to his own designs, free of university bureaucrats.

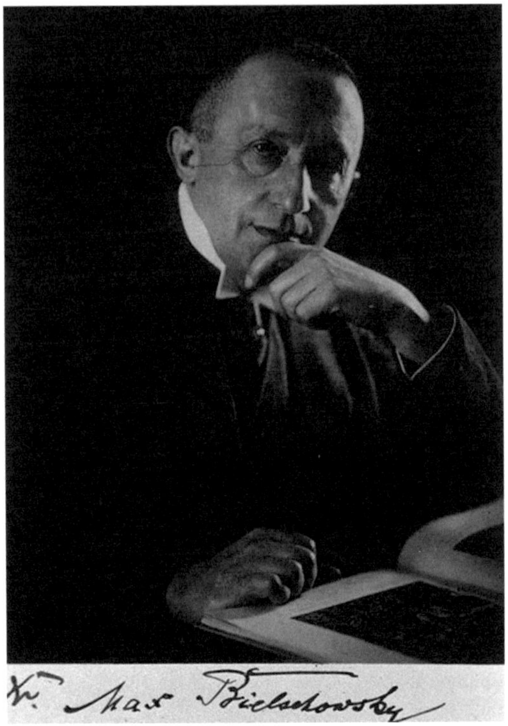

FIGURE 1.5: Max Bielschowsky (1869–1940) was a Polish neuropathologist credited with the development of the Bielschowsky silver impregnation technique.

The historical record nevertheless has suffered some decay over time. As remarkable as Alzheimer's observations were, and as much as the changes themselves did represent a springboard toward lesion-based biological analysis of chronic disease, they are overstated in terms of attribution; this overstatement ironically occurs with greater regularity now than at any other time in history. It is customary now, for example, to find historical accounts of Alois Alzheimer's Description of Auguste D., along with his putative original observations of the neuropathological lesions within her cerebral cortex, among introductory remarks in contemporary discussions on Alzheimer's Disease (AD). Invariably, the senile plaque is noted first and attributed to Alzheimer as a landmark pathological correlation. The neurofibrillary tangle is often, although not always, discussed, and then almost invariably subsequent to the mention of the plaque. For example, in "Reimagining Alzheimer's Disease—an Age-based Hypothesis," a biochemist writes:

> *"In 1906, Alois Alzheimer reported the first description of the dementing illness that now bears his name. He documented the progression of symptoms that beset a farmer's wife Auguste D., as her mental status deteriorated through a complex series of behavioral and cognitive changes that left*

her aggressive, delusional, and unable to recall recent events. After her death Alzheimer's Drew on his interest in the emerging techniques of histochemistry. He stained sections from the autopsied brain and discovered the presence of "miliar foci, which are caused by deposition of a pecular substance in the cortex" (now recognized as the neuritic or senile plaque). He also reported "very peculiar changes in the neurofibrils" (now recognized as compared helical filaments or tangles). By concerning himself with the structure of the diseased brain and the abnormal deposits that he found, he was among the early pioneers whose studies link brain structure to function." [8]

In "Alzheimer's Disease," a clinician writes:

"The description of the clinico-pathological syndrome by the Bavarian psychiatrist, Alois Alzheimer, in 1906 established a neuropathological phenotype that has enabled considerable diagnostic specificity, although until recently only at the end of the patient's life. The microscopic lesions that Alzheimer called attention to—senile (amyloid) plaques and neurofibrillary tangles—have also provided a crucial starting point for approaching molecular pathogenesis. Indeed, the principal reasons that substantial progress toward deciphering the disease has accrued are its high prevalence and the robustness of its histological signature." [9]

The picture being painted by AD scholars as they invoke the seminal observations of Alzheimer is clear: Alois Alzheimer's identification of hallmark lesions in the brain of Auguste D., altered the direction of biomedical research into AD and aging, and profoundly influenced the pathway toward understanding the disease process, and ultimately, successful intervention. His observations were both cunning and fortuitous, particularly in light of the amyloid cascade concept later elaborated, as without these seminal observations by Alzheimer, the concept would simply not exist or would have been substantially delayed, and the scientific community in their ignorance might have followed an ill-fated path away from the amyloid cascade. Such a picture is both historically inaccurate, and scientifically flawed, possibly in the extreme.

While there is no doubt that lesion identification opened an avenue for research (the process of clinico-pathological correlation has led to more advances in medicine than any other single discipline), it is less clear that the accumulation of copious knowledge of lesions and their histogenesis has led to an improved understanding of disease etiology, and less clear still that we are in any way poised for meaningful intervention [10, 11]. Equating lesion with etiopathogenesis is a dubious proposition, as the study of neurodegeneration has shown over the last several decades, and it may well be that the talents of countless investigators and the expenditure of boundless public treasure has been exhausted in an attempt to prove that lesion constituents are toxic [10]. To his credit, Alzheimer himself was remarkably more circumspect. One quote in particular is noteworthy, as it still holds, despite extensive efforts to prove:

"although one might be tempted to do so, one cannot relate plaques to fibrillary change and vice versa." [4]

Max Bielschowsky, who developed the techniques necessary to make the observation of Alzheimer and his contemporaries possible, was similarly measured about the significance of pathological changes in chronic disease:

"Such observations demonstrate to us that we may employ the conception of specificity in the histopathology of ganglion cells only with the greatest caution. It must be emphasized once again that pathological cell types give us no direct indications for a precise diagnosis, but only reveal that in the nervous system pathological processes have been taking place. They indicate whether these processes are progressing more or less rapidly and whether they tend to destroy the cell life or only exert a passing influence. Consequently cell pictures are of value as indicators of pathological reactions only in the general sense. Moreover, it must be remembered that they may be considered only partial manifestations of processes involving the whole tissue complex. The changes of neuroglia, of the circulatory apparatus and connective tissue are of equal importance in the formation of our judgments of the etiological relationship between occasional anatomical findings and the associated clinical picture." [12]

It may also surprise the reader to know that Alzheimer was not the first to describe senile plaques. Nor indeed was he the first to link senile plaques to dementia [13]. While this may at first appear to deplete the significance of the original case as a seminal moment in scientific progress, it also encourages a recollection of the naming of the disease, its relationship to aging, and the justification of a new entity in the first place.

The more complete historical record indicates that between 1890 and 1892, Blocq and Marinesco (Figure 1.6) identified plaques in the brains of epileptic patients at Salpetriere Hospital in Paris [14]. The lesions, which they termed "nodules of nevroglial sclerosis," were found in various layers of the cerebral cortex and measured about 60 microns in diameter, making it reasonably clear that they were describing today's senile plaques. Prior to this work, Beljahow described neurodegenerative changes in senile dementia which, although somewhat vague, raise the possibility that he described both senile plaques and neurofibrillary tangles [15], and this nearly 20 years prior to Alzheimer's Description of Auguste D.

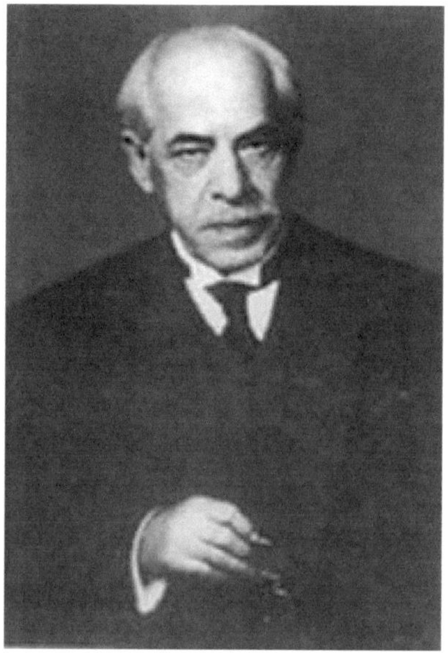

FIGURE 1.6: Gheorghe Marinesco, the famous neurohistologist and founder of the Romanian School of Neurology, may have been the first to describe senile plaques, along with his associate, Paul Blocq, in 1892 [14].

In 1898, Emil Redlich (Figure 1.7), at the University of Vienna, described 'miliare Skelerose' in two patients with senile dementia clinically [16], and was the first to use the term "plaque" to describe the structures. He identified plaques using carmine red in one of the patients who was 78 years old and suffered from severe dementia, and suggested that plaques were most likely of glial origin. Interestingly, Redlich reflected on whether the lesions were a primary event or a reactive phenomenon, a debate that is ongoing at present and not at all resolved.

In 1906, Koichi Miyake from the Psychiatric Clinic of Tokyo University, who had trained in Vienna, reported on the changes in the aging cerebral cortex [17]. Miyake studied 25 brains, of which four suffered from dementia, and of these, two demonstrated senile plaques. Like Redlich, Miyake believed the plaques to be of glial origin.

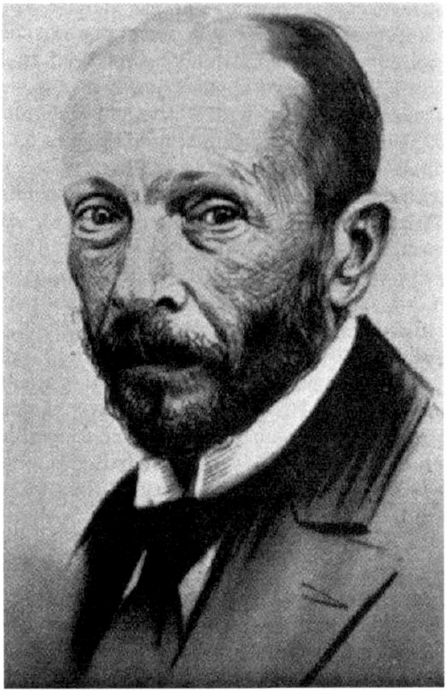

FIGURE 1.7: Emil Redlich (1866–1930) described and even used the term "plaque" in patients with senile dementia nearly a decade prior to Alzheimer's Description of Auguste D. [170].

Whereas Alzheimer may be credited with the first description of the neurofibrillary tangle, Oskar Fischer was the first to identify and characterize the neuritic plaque, and he did so in extraordinary detail (Figure 1.8) [18]. In his 1907 paper, Fischer studied autopsy brains in 16 cases of senile dementia, using the recently developed Bielschowsky silver impregnation technique [19]. He noted plaques in 12 of 16 of the senile dementia cases, which were not seen in cases of psychosis, neurosyphilis, or controls. This led to the elaboration of a temporal staging sequence in his 1910 paper with both qualitative and quantitative differences [20]. Importantly, included with the plaques in intermediate stages were distended, club-shaped neurites, the basis of the modern day neuritic plaque. Overall, the plaques ranged in size from 10 microns to 120 microns, with better developed plaques containing a dense core of material surrounded by a radiating corona of finer fibrillar material, so much so as to resemble sulfur granules of actinomycosis (*Aktinomyesdruse*). Fischer further made reference to what is now known as cerebral amyloid angiopathy.

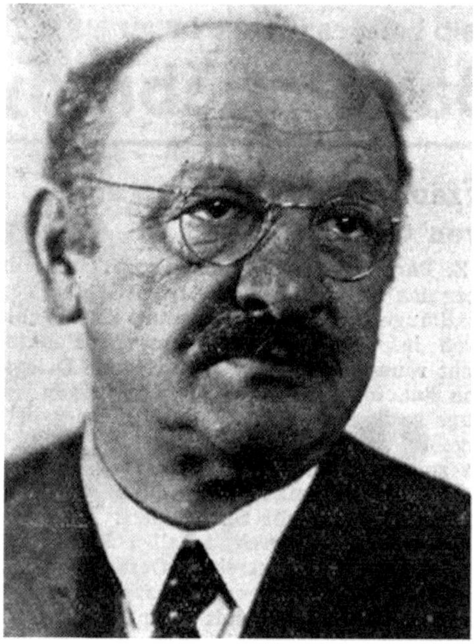

FIGURE 1.8: Oskar Fischer (1876-1942) was both a pioneering and tragic figure in the history of neuroscience. Fischer was the first to describe the neuritic plaque, now recognized as the signature lesion of Alzheimer's Disease, which he did in copious detail. Fischer, however, maintained an association between neuritic plaques and presbyophrenia, the latter an antiquated term referring to confabulations, marked memory impairment, hyperactivity, disorientation, elevated mood, and preserved social graces [200]. Fischer was arrested by the Gestapo in 1941 and taken to the Small Fortress in Terazìn in northwestern Bohemia, and died of an apparent heart attack in February 1942 [18].

It is interesting to note the description in English of plaque pathology by an Alzheimer contemporary Solomon C. Fuller, M.D., of the Pathological Laboratory, Westborough State Hospital, published in the *American Journal of Insanity* in 1911 [21]. In his study, Dr. Solomon details the late 19th-century and early 20th-century literature of so-called miliary plaques. The finding of plaques by Redlich in 1898 is highlighted as a critical observation, whereas the work of Blocq and Marinesco six years prior was also well known. Studies from a number of other eminent researchers of the day, including Perusini, Heubner, Simchowicz, Fischer, Oppenheim, Bonfiglio, Barrett, Herxheimer, and Gierlich are all mentioned, some indicating a clear association between plaques and senile dementia, others emphasizing the identification of plaques with advanced age, and still others (e.g., Fischer) emphasizing a relationship with more specific clinical signs such as presbyophrenia. Alzheimer is mentioned as well, but only in the sense that his two cases were atypical in their early onset, possible advanced pathology, and possible focal neurological signs. Neurofibrillary tangles are mentioned in passing, as a finding of Alzheimer but which was noted by other investigators around the same time frame. Since the original illustrations NFTs were not published by Alzheimer until he reported his two early onset cases in 1910, it may be argued whether Alzheimer should even be credited with the first description of NFTs. Indeed, the combination of plaques and tangles with dementia were reported by Bonfiglio in 1908 [22], Perusini in 1909 [23], Sarteschi in 1909 [24], and Barrett in 1911.

The reality of Alzheimer's notoriety that continues to the present day, however, probably has more to do with the eponym created by Kraepelin in the 8th edition of his textbook of psychiatry [5]. In this text, Kraepelin introduces a new condition, Alzheimer's Disease, as a form of atypical dementia with some clinical and pathological overlap with senile dementia, but with a younger age at onset, tendency for focal signs, and a tendency for severe pathology. Kraepelin justifies the new condition as follows, once again highlighting that the atypicality rested more in the clinical presentation than the histopathological changes:

> *"Although the anatomical findings would suggest the assumption that this is a matter of particularly severe form of senile dementia, to some extent this is contradicted by the circumstances that the illness at times already begins at the end of the 40th year."* [2]

One objective advance since 1906 has been the recognition of familial disease linked to germline mutation in the gene for amyloid precursor protein (APP), presenilin 1 (PS1), and presenilin 2 (PS2). Since patients with one of these mutations tend to have early onset disease, it may be argued with some conviction that Auguste D. or perhaps Alzheimer's second patient, Johann F., may have had germline mutations, and that the novelty of this new so-called Alzheimer's Disease was its familial nature, resulting in early onset. Indeed, a presenilin 2 mutation was initially suspected, based on a recent study identifying a presenilin 2 N141I mutation in German's of Volga ancestry, like Auguste D. [25]. This was refuted by genetic analysis of tissue section from Auguste D.'s brain [26], although a more recent study by the same group identified a possible F176L presenilin 1 mutation [27]. Pedigree analysis of Johann F. also shows a suggestion of autosomal dominant disease [28], although no mutation was characterized. Both Auguste D. and Johann F. were found to be homozygous ε3 at the apolipoprotein E allele.

In short, it is interesting to note the subtle distortion of not only the science of Alzheimer's Disease since its description over 100 years ago, but also the historical record. Alzheimer's Disease was named, and its existence justified, not because of the identification of pathological correlates to senile dementia. Indeed, plaques and their association with senile dementia were well known some years before Auguste D.'s description. What made Alzheimer's Disease novel was the young age at onset and its association with atypical clinical signs. As one looks back, it appears that Alzheimer's Disease was familial early onset disease of today, and senile dementia then, was sporadic Alzheimer's Disease of today. It might also be frankly admitted that the eagerness with which pathological lesions are attributed to Alzheimer in recent years has at its roots in an affective desire to promote lesion constituents as causative, targetable phenomena, which in turn highlights the progress of the last 30 years and serves as a prelude to the anticipated success of lesion targeting. The fact that proof of concept has been achieved, i.e., that lesions and their proteins have been removed from diseased brains during life [29], with no measureable change in the downward cognitive trajectory, has not also not resulted in a measureable change in the extent to which the hypothesis is (or more accurately, is not) questioned. It thus appears that efforts in science in the 21st century might benefit substantially from more individuals like Alois Alzheimer, who embraced objectivity, and did not have a personal, financial, or emotional stake in the material success an idea.

CHAPTER 2
Plaques

2.1 PATHOLOGY

It should be stated at the outset that plaques of any form are specific only for some length of elapsed time, roughly measured in decades, and are not specific to any disease process, clinical state, or cognitive trajectory. While it may be said that the larger the number of plaques in the neocortex, the more likely it is that the affected individual showed cognitive deterioration during life [30], even this relationship all but ceases to exist in the very old [31]. This set of empirical facts is often set aside, and set aside more often now than any other time in history, probably because dominant schools of thought require pathogenicity of plaques [32]. Without such a requirement, the objective-minded neurobiologist might frankly admit that, for practical purposes, no more is known about the origin of plaques today than in 1892, aside perhaps from rare Mendelian conditions with known pathogenic mutations. Nor is the weak correlation between plaque quantity and dementia better characterized.

Nevertheless, since Blocq and Marinesco first noted "nodules of nevroglial sclerosis" in an elderly epileptic patient over 120 years ago, plaques and their constituents have been studied extensively. Bielschowsky silver impregnation staining was the first technical advance that highlighted plaques much better than previously available dyes. Interestingly, the Bielschowsky technique had its origin in the production of mirrors based on its use of the silver diamine complex that precipitates on the interface between a glass surface and the solution. The initial application to tissue was improved by Bielschowsky by incubating formalin fixed tissues in silver nitrate prior to the silver diamine, along with pretreatment with pyridine [33]. The most commonly used and arguably most reproducible modification of the Bielschowsky technique is that proposed by Yamamoto and Hirano [34], which employs the usual silver nitrate-ammoniacal silver steps, followed by another ammoniacal silver step in the developer. If done properly, Bielschowsky silver methods highlight not only senile plaques, but neurofibrillary tangles in AD and Pick bodies in Pick disease while normal tissues remain.

While a seemingly singular "hallmark" lesion, the plaque actually represents a spectrum of changes and morphologies, which has in turn prompted morphologic subclassification. As a result, the nosology of plaques is somewhat confusing, overlapping, and imprecisely correlated with disease as a function of subtype. They generally measure 40–60 μm in diameter, although some may be smaller, while others may measure up to 200 μm (Table 2.1).

TABLE 2.1: Plaque nosology

Amyloid plaque	Congo red-positive plaque
Aβ plaque	Any plaque with Aβ immunoreactivity
Senile plaque	Ill-defined term for a number of plaque subtypes
Diffuse plaque	Amorphous Aβ immunoreactivity, lacking fibrillarity
Primitive plaque	Aβ plaque with no amyloid core and ill-defined neuritic component
Cotton wool plaque	Aβ plaque with no fibrillary amyloid or neurites, often in PS1-linked AD
Cored plaque	Aβ plaque with discrete amyloid core
Compact plaque	Synonymous with cored plaque
Neuritic plaque	Plaque with amyloid core and dystrophic, often tau-positive neurites
Mature plaque	Neuritic or cored plaque
Classic plaque	Neuritic plaque
Lake-like plaque	large Aβ deposit, often in the parvocellular layer of the presubiculum
Fleecy plaque	Loosely tectured Aβ plaque found in the entorhinal cortex
Band-like plaque	Subpial Aβ deposit, often with adjacent amyloid angiopathy

Divry in 1927 demonstrated an affinity of plaques for Congo red, indicating a component of amyloid, and leading to the generic term "amyloid plaque" [35] (Figure 2.1). This has progressed to a slightly more modern term, the amyloid-β (Aβ) plaque, given the protein consistent of a major amyloid species within plaques. On the other hand, plaques may be comprised solely of diffuse, non-fibrillar Aβ, identifiable by immunohistochemistry, generally negative for Congo red, variably detectable with thioflavin S (Figure 2.1), and variably detectable with silver impregnation such as the Bielschowsky. Such lesions are generally referred to as "diffuse plaques" (DP). DP appear first in the neocortex in young individuals, making it especially difficult to relate their presence to disease, and especially easy to discount them as "age related." DP have therefore been regarded as "non-pathogenic," marginally pathological, or decorative phenomena. The appearance of DP both in time and space raises the issue of kinetics of DP progression over time, although there is no proof of chronology at present.

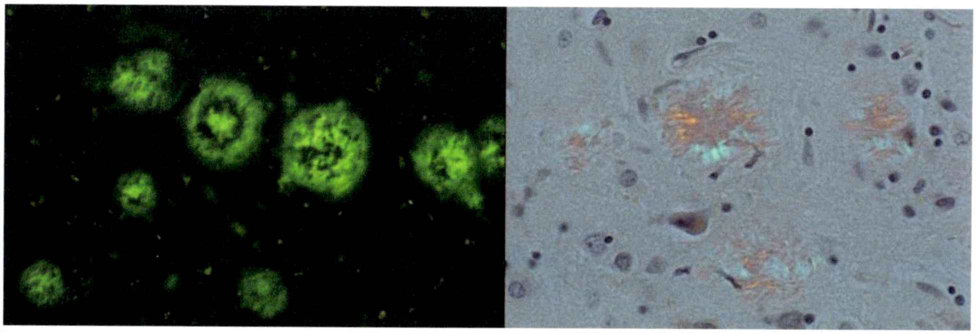

FIGURE 2.1: Thioflavin S (left) is a commonly used histochemical technique for demonstrating plaque pathology as well as cerebral amyloid angiophathy. Congo red with apple-green birefringence (right) indicates the presence of fibrillar amyloid with increased β-sheet content, although this technique is less sensitive than Aβ immunohistochemistry, and therefore less commonly used. Congo red also stains neurofibrillary tangles, which led early investigators to speculate on its similarity to senile plaque amyloid and its subcellular location (intracellular versus extracellular).

While impossible to study in humans, it is reasonable to speculate that some DP have the capacity to mature into better developed structural lesions [36]. Their appearance in Down syndrome brains early in life prior to the invariable, neuritic pathology later on, suggests that the DP is a precursor to the NP. For now, it suffices to distinguish Aβ plaques, which are immunohistochemically detectable deposits of Aβ in any form, from DP, which are non-fibrillar, Congo red-negative, thioflavin-negative deposits of Aβ, from amyloid plaques, which would be any form of plaque which is Congo red- or Thioflavin-positive. Also noteworthy is that DP as detected by anti-Aβ immunohistochemistry may occasionally occupy an exceptionally large volume, exceeding several microns, referred to as "lake-like" Aβ deposits; these are typically seen in the parvocellular layer of the presubiculum. So-called fleecy Aβ deposits are sometimes seen in the entorhinal cortex, whereas band-like subpial Aβ deposits may be found, with or without adjacent blood vessels affected by cerebral amyloid angiopathy [37]. The pathogenic significance of lake-like, fleecy, and band-like Aβ deposits has not been particularly well studied, although they do indicate a level of heterogeneity that might be taken into account with the use of generic terms like "senile plaque" (Figure 2.2).

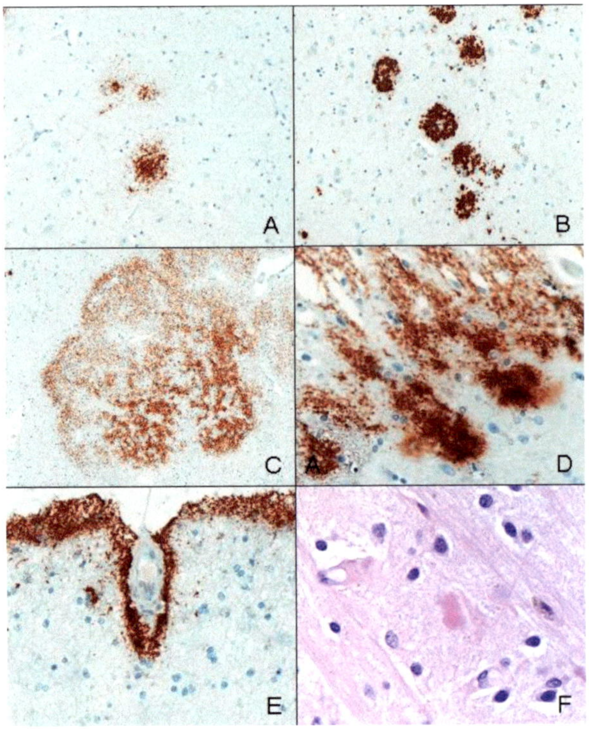

FIGURE 2.2: A number of morphological subtypes of Aβ plaques have no pathogenic relevance in the literature to date. Among these are diffuse plaques (A), primitive plaques (B), lake-like plaques of the parvocellular layer of the presubiculum (C), fleecy plaques of the entorhinal cortex (D), subpial band-like deposits (E), and discrete parenchymal deposits of amyloid (mature, cored, or "burned out" plaques) with little or no tissue reaction (F). Monoclonal antibody 4G8, which recognized the mid-molecular epitope of Aβ is used in figures 10A through 10E.

Next in the morphological sequence is a lesser-mentioned plaque type referred as the "primitive plaque." A primitive plaque would have detectable, somewhat spheroid deposits that may be detectable by Congo red or thioflavin S, but have poorly developed dystrophic neurites, and lack an amyloid core. Whether the primitive plaque represents a morphological progression from the DP, while seemingly reasonable, is controversial [36].

The association between advanced age/senility with plaques dates essentially to their original description, hence the use of the term "senile plaque" (SP), which loosely refers to any of a number of plaque subtypes. Since they were initially described with the help of Bielschowsky silver technique, senile plaques are probably synonymous with Aβ plaques, and therefore could correspond to diffuse, compact, neuritic, cored or mature, and/or "cotton wool" subtypes.

A less common but also long known plaque subtype is the "cotton wool" plaque, the name referring to the loosely tectured appearance regardless of technique used to identify them (routine dyes such as hematoxylin and eosin, Bielschowsky, immunohistochemistry), although they are readily identified even on routine hematoxylin and eosin preparations. Cotton wool plaques may be observed in advanced age and sporadic AD. The descriptive term dates back to Oskar Fischer [18]. They were generally ignored as a significant or distinguishing finding for many decades, until they were observed as a dominant finding in some cases of familial early AD with presenilin-1 mutations [38]. Cotton wool plaques are said to lack fibrillary amyloid and dystrophic neurites, although contain amorphous collections of protein, much of which is comprised of Aβ. Little is known about their histogenesis and why they can be comprised of rather dense collections of Aβ and still lack biochemically definable amyloid and phosphorylated tau. While prominent in familial AD with PS1 mutation, cotton wool plaques are not limited to this condition. [39]

In contrast to the cotton wool plaque that lacks fibrillar amyloid, the so-called "cored" plaque may be comprised solely of fibrillar amyloid. Cored plaques, like other plaque subtypes, are common in both aging and AD, and are somewhat loosely defined in terms of a size and associated pathology. A dense core of Aβ in the absence of dystrophic neurites or reactive glia indicates a purely cored plaque, while dense plaque cores may also occur in association with dystrophic neurites, including tau positive dystrophic neurites. For obscure reasons, "pure" cored plaques, sometimes referred to as "mature" plaques, or "burned out" plaques, i.e., rounded accumulation of fibrillary, Congo red positive amyloid with virtually no associated pathology or inflammatory reaction, are found in specific neuroanatomical sites, including the cerebellar Purkinje and granular cell layers, the globus pallidus, primary cortical areas including area 17 of the visual cortex and the pericentral region. This is in contrast to diffuse, primitive, and neuritic plaques (see below), which predominate in multimodal association cortices associated with cognition and executive functions, as well as limbic cortices. The existence of pure cored plaques, i.e., parenchymal amyloid with no associated neuritic or inflammatory reaction, serves as a reminder of the heterogeneity of plaques in general, and may render simplistic the linear constructs that relate proteins to general neurotoxicity.

The plaque subtype that has attracted the most attention in the literature is the neuritic plaque (NP), also known as the classic plaque (Figure 2.3). As noted above, the description of the NP dates back to Oskar Fischer in 1907, around the same time that Alzheimer's Described neurofibrillary tangles [19, 20]. NP according to Fischer were characterized by miliary foci within or near which were found Bielschowsky-impregnable, club-shaped, swollen neurofibrils, known as dystrophic neurites in modern terminology. The appeal of the neuritic plaque over other plaque subtypes rests in the fact that it combines both plaque pathology and neurofibrillary pathology. As such, they seemingly encompass more completely the neurodegenerative process, and although any lesion detected at autopsy is static by definition, NPs are often looked upon as a mechanistically dynamic lesion, embodying a temporal sequence of Aβ overproduction, extracellular Aβ deposition, Aβ fibrillization into biochemically detectable amyloid, neuroinflammation with microglia, and ultimately Aβ-mediated neuritic damage with accumulation of phospho-tau within dystrophic neurites [30].

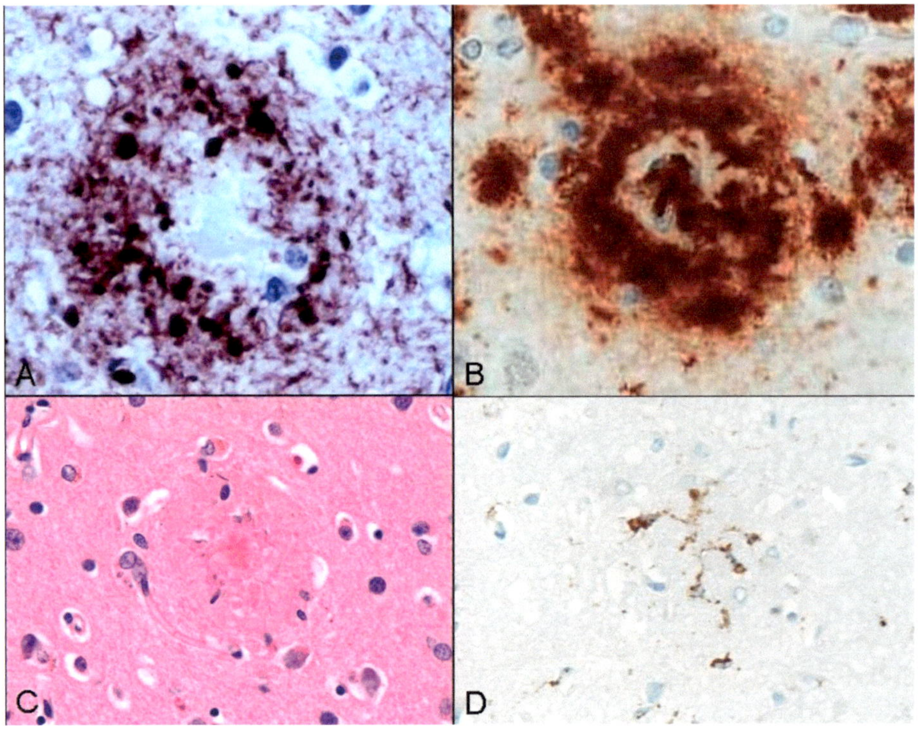

FIGURE 2.3: The neuritic plaque is widely regarded as the plaque subtype with the most pathogenic significance, since it encompasses deposits of both Aβ and phosphorylated tau. The tissue reaction comprised of dystrophic neurites, gliosis, and neuroinflammation with microglial activation. Monoclonal antibody AT8, a particularly robust phospho-tau antibody recognizing phospho-serine at residue 202 and phospho-threonine at residue 205, shows the neuritic component of the neuritic plaque in Figure 2.3A. Aβ immunohistochemistry in Figure 2.3B shows a neuritic plaque. With careful observation at high magnification, neuritic plaques may be apparent with routine dyes such as hematolyxin and eosin (C), while CD68 immunohistochemistry (D) shows microglial cells within the plaque.

Given the requirement of the dystrophic neurite in order to define a plaque as neuritic, it is tempting to also require the presence of phosphorylated tau within a plaque as part of the definition. While this is often the case, particularly in neocortical association areas, dystrophic neurites may be Bielschowsky silver-positive and yet fail to accumulate phosphorylated tau [40], suggesting that the neuritic abnormalities predate tau accumulation. To complicate the issue further, ultrastructural studies demonstrate neurites even in association with diffuse Aβ deposits [41]. In either case, some neuropathologists believe that the Bielschowsky silver technique, is a more sensitive indicator of NP, which is in turn the explanation for why this arcane histologic technique which substantially predates the advent of the central dogma of molecular biology is still recommended in modern consensus guidelines for AD diagnosis at autopsy [42].

In summary, plaques are heterogeneous in terms of size, morphology, presence, and extent of associated structural alterations, protein constituents, cellular constituents, and clinical correlates. All plaque subtypes may be observed in cognitively intact individuals, whereas an absence of plaques is invariable in young individuals. The differences in pathology between cognitively intact and clinically demented individuals are largely quantitative and become increasingly blurred with advancing age, as discussed below. The tendency for neuroscientists to view the neuritic plaque as the embodiment of disease pathogenesis, including temporal sequences of proteinopathies, is remarkable, particularly in light of our limited knowledge of temporal kinetics of plaques *in vivo*. We instead favor the view that plaques represent a complex response to age and/or disease, which explains the overall lack of specificity, variable region specificity, and our inability to impact the disease process by plaque removal.

2.2 THE PURIFICATION OF AMYLOID

George Glenner and Caine Wong provided a landmark study and one of the most highly cited papers in biomedical science, in *Biochemical and Biophysical Research Communications* in 1984 [43]. Interestingly, the specific rationale involved the study of amyloidosis, drawing parallels to known amyloid proteins at that time, with the ultimate hope of developing a serum diagnostic test for AD. It is also interesting to note that a major precept of the study, that "cerebrovascular amyloidosis is seen only in Alzheimer's Disease, adult Down's syndrome individuals, and a familial Icelandic cerebrovascular amyloidosis syndrome," is fundamentally incorrect in that sporadic cerebral amyloid angiopathy commonly occurs with age in the absence of AD or dementia (Figure 2.4). Nevertheless, the study was ground breaking at the time, as it involved the purification of pathological lesions from the human brain.

In this study, Glenner and Wong stripped leptomeningeal blood vessels from human brain, removed gross gray matter contaminants, and homogenized the tissue at 12,500 x g for 60 minutes. The top layer of the pellet, which was demonstrably enriched with amyloid as shown by Congo red staining, was homogenized in buffer and placed back in solution. After further digestion with collagenase, the amyloid solution was ultra-centrifuged, and the resulting pellet detergent extracted. G-100 Sephadex column chromatography was then performed, the protein peak pooled and dialyzed, lyophilized and stored dessicated at -70 C. High performance liquid chromatography of the peak fractions of the Sephadex columns was then undertaken, protein peaks further pooled and lyophilized, amino acids analyzed, and finally subjected to automated amino acid sequencing to 24 residues. The results indicated the following peptide: NH2-Asp-Ala-Glu-Phe-Arg-His-Asp-Ser-Gly-Tyr-Gln-Val-His-His-Gln-Lys-Leu-Val-Phe-Phe-Ala-Glu-Asp-Val-COOH.

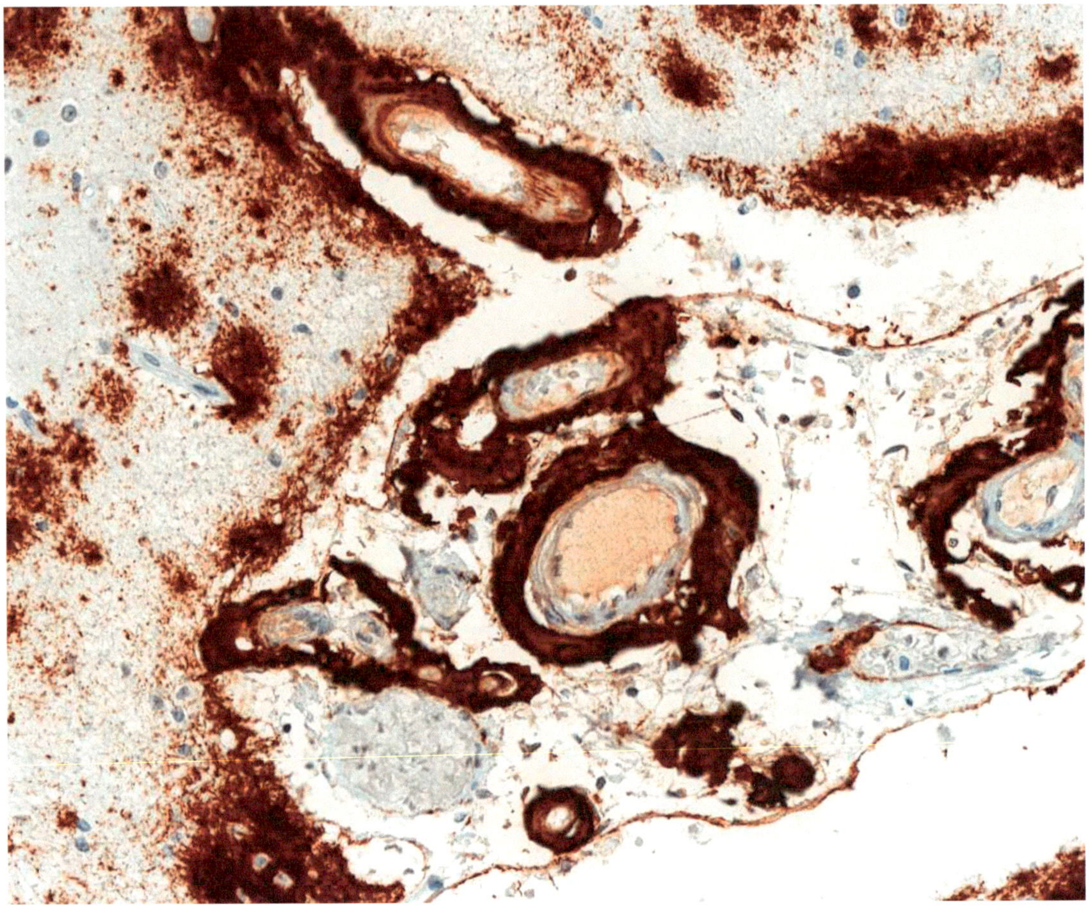

FIGURE 2.4: Aβ (4G8) immunohistochemistry demonstrates dense accumulation of Aβ within blood vessel walls in cerebral amyloid angiopathy. Cerebral amyloid angiopathy is the most common cause of lobar intracerebral hemorrhage in individuals over the age of 65 and is frequently seen in the absence of cognitive impairment [200].

The same investigators then performed the same experiments using cerebrovascular tissue obtained at autopsy from two subjects, age 61 and 62, affected by Down syndrome, finding a nearly identical 24 amino acid peptide, differing only in the presence of Glu instead of Gln at position

11. The protein, referred to as beta-2 because of the highest peak on HPLC, was not felt to be homologous to the serum protein gamma trace found in cerebrovascular vessels of patients with Icelandic hereditary amyloid angiopathy (later characterized as a cystatin C-related familial cerebral amyloid). The results were further encouraging for the development of a diagnostic test, as well as animal models with a molecular-based construct. Given the near-identical biochemical similarity in beta proteins between AD and Down syndrome, chromosome 21 was immediately suggested as the localization of the gene encoding the β protein. Shortly thereafter, investigators from several laboratories used oligonucleotide probes corresponding to the amino acid sequence of the purified protein to isolate a cDNA clone corresponding to the β-amyloid precursor protein (AβPP) on the long arm of chromosome 21 [44–46], and metabolic pathway was born.

While AD research in the mid-1980s was expanding exponentially with the identification and characterization of Aβ and AβPP, it is interesting to note that the foundation of the entire area of investigation was based on the concept that cerebral amyloid angiopathy was disease specific and not a reactive process. Nevertheless, the extent of new knowledge of lesion constituents and their similarities in AD and Down syndrome, provided sufficient momentum to discard in wholesale fashion the idea that Aβ, either in cerebral blood vessels or neuritic plaques, was neither diagnostic of AD nor even a marker of dementia. This era in science was indeed a tribute to the power of central dogma of molecular biology and the ease with which whole organism, chronic, and highly complex disease processes such as sporadic AD are attributed to single small molecules, produced physiologically and with intact primary structure. Even as far back as the 1984 landmark paper by Glenner and Wong, the allure of a potential serum diagnostic test was palpable, as was the drive toward animal modeling, with little regard for human relevance. Both of these goals continue as of this writing with unabated enthusiasm, in the form of the search for biomarkers and expansion of transgenic animal constructs. Yet 30 years later, no serum diagnostic test is on the horizon, and no animal model that has reportedly shown promise in preclinical studies has translated to positive data in clinical trials [10].

2.3 AMYLOID-B PROTEIN PRECURSOR

On the other hand, knowledge of Aβ and AβPP processing is copious (Figure 2.5), and beyond the scope of the present work. Briefly, the AβPP gene is localized to chromosome 21 at 21q21.2 [44, 47]. It is encoded by 19 exons, while exons 16 and 17 encode the Aβ amyloid peptide [48, 49]. Three major splicing variants have been identified containing the Aβ amyloid sequence, containing 695, 751, and 770 residues respectively. AβPP is a component of cellular metabolism in general, as it is expressed in all tissues, all nucleated cells, and platelets. Moreover, the AβPP promoter lacks a TATA box and contains a high CG content, two features of so-called housekeeping genes. On the other hand, mRNA for the 695 amino acid splice variant, or AβPP695, is the major APP species found in the

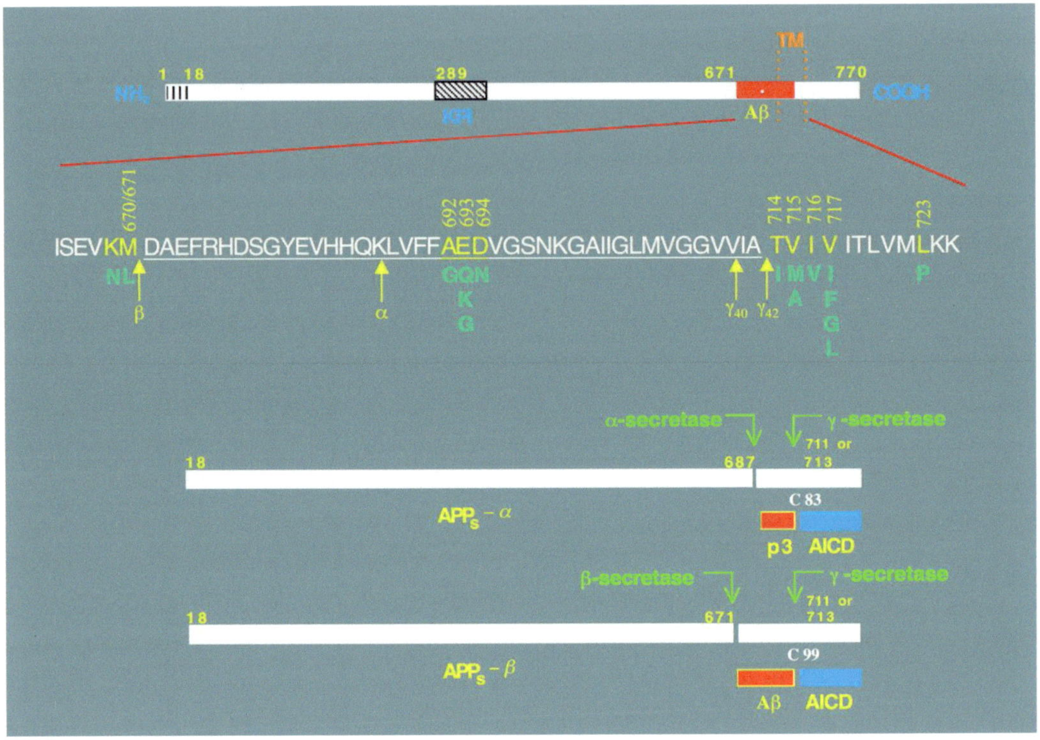

FIGURE 2.5: A schematic diagram depicts the major biological processing of amylid precursor protein. Three major splicing variants have been identified containing the Aβ amyloid sequence, containing 695, 751, and 770 residues respectively, although mRNA for the the 695 amino acid splice variant, or AβPP695, is the major APP species found in the brain. β is a type 1 transmembrane protein with general housekeeping properties, a relatively short cytosolic component, and a relatively lengthy extracellular component. Exon 7, codes for the 57-amino-acid Kunitz type protease inhibitor (KPI) domain. Full length AβPP may be cleaved with α- or β-secretase, liberating the extracellular N-terminal AβPP of about 687 and 671 amino acids respectively, with retained C-terminal membrane bound fragments of 83 and 99 amino acids (C83, C89), respectively. Production of full length Aβ requires β-secretase cleavage, considered the rate limiting step for Aβ synthesis, followed by "promiscuous" γ-secretase cleavage, yielding Aβ and the AβPP intracellular C-terminal domain (AICD). α-secretase cleavage instead results in a truncated Aβ fragment referred to as P3 (with loss of the metal binding portion of Aβ and retention of the amyloidogenic component), and a longer AICD. Germline mutations in various codons in the AβPP gene are depicted; the majority occurs within or near the Aβ region. Both the P3 and Aβ pathways are physiologic processes throughout life.

brain. The AβPP751 and AβPP770 mRNA both contain exon 7, which codes for a 57-amino-acid domain with sequence homology to Kunitz type protease inhibitor (KPI) and is referred to as the KPI domain [50–52]. Exon 8 encodes for a 19-amino-acid domain with homology to the MRC OX-2 antigen [53]. A number of other less common splice variants have also been described, with alternative splicing of exons 7, 8, and 15. The amino acid sequence predicts that AβPP is a type-I oriented (alpha-helical present in the inner membranes of bacterial cells or the plasma membrane of eukaryotes, and sometimes in the outer membranes), with a single transmembrane domain near the carboxy terminus within the cytosol, and amino terminus within the extracellular space. AβPP undergoes a number of post-translational modifications, including N- and O-glycosylation, tyrosine sulfation, and phosphorylation. However, only about 10% of AβPP reaches the cell surface, while the bulk of AβPP localizes to the golgi and trans-golgi network. AβPP that is not secreted is rapidly internalized due to its so-called YENPTY internalization motif, near the C-terminus. AβPP then enters the endocytic pathway, where it may be recycled to the plasma membrane or degraded. The YENPTY and adjacent regions appear to serve as binding sites for many cytosolic adaptors (Fe65, Mint 2, Mint 3, etc.), which appear to regulate amyloidogenic processing via β- and γ-secretases in the endocyic pathway [54].

AβPP is proteolytically processed by the action of three enzymes, termed secretases, referring to the secreted nature of the cleaved products [54]. The three most studied secretases are referred to as α-secretase, β-secretase, and γ-secretase. The actions of α-secretase and β-secretase are mutually exclusive, such that two overall pathways are possible, commonly called non-amyloidogenic and amyloidogenic respectively, although it should be kept in mind that both processes occur throughout life, and that even the amyloidogenic pathway proceeds for decades with no detectable deposits of Aβ within the brain by immunohistochemistry. α-secretase cleavage appears to occur principally at the cell surface, while β-secretase cleavage occurs in the endocytic pathway (Figure 2.6).

Aβ is produced in the amyloidogenic pathway by the consecutive action of β- and γ-secretase. As Aβ occupies portions of the transmembrane domain as well as extracellular domain, γ-secretase cleaves AβPP within the tranmembrane domain, and β- secretase cleaves within the extracellular domain. Both enzymes have received considerable attention because of their role in generating Aβ, and warrant brief discussion.

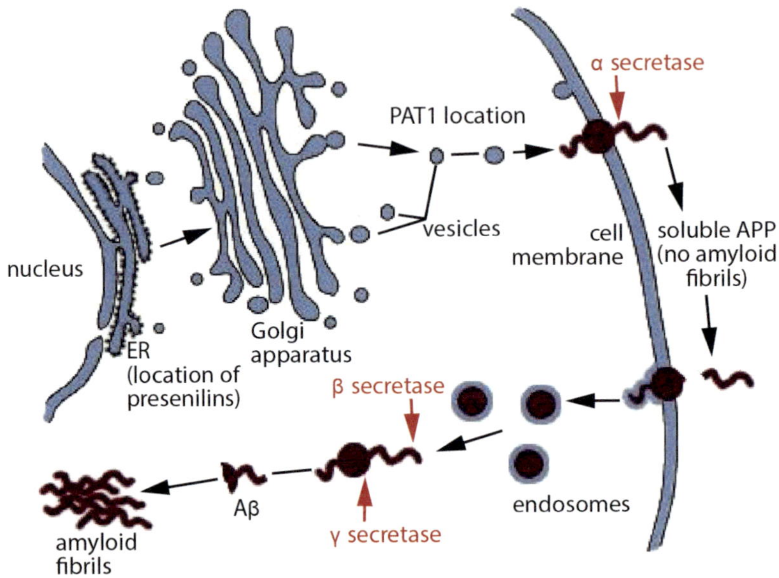

FIGURE 2.6: Cellular schematic diagram of AβPP metabolism indicates that α-secretase tends to occur at the cell surface, while β-secretase activity occurs in the endocytic pathway. The potential pathogenic significance of this feature of the cell biology has been addressed by numerous studies, although the normal physiological role of AβPP metabolism remains largely a mystery.

2.4 SECRETASES

2.4.1 BACE-1

Early cell culture studies indicated the presence of a membrane-bound 99 residue C terminal fragment of AβPP, and a secreted AβPP fragment [55]. Initially, this so-called β-secretase was indirectly implicated because of the nature of AβPP fragments identified. Early studies were directed at cathepsin D, but this was disproven by experimental knockout studies. Further studies differed on whether β-secretase cleaved AβPP during endocytic processing versus extracellularly when AβPP reached the cell surface. In 1999, several groups reported that β-secretase was a novel integral membrane aspartyl protease, which had not been previously identified in humans [56–60]. Among the groups identifying β-secretase, one in particular isolated β-secretase cDNA in an expression screen for cDNAs that had demonstrable increases in Aβ production. The group coined the enzyme BACE, for β (Beta) site AβPP-Cleaving Enzyme, which has since been broadly adopted [59]. Not surprisingly, BACE homologues were recognized shortly thereafter, in particular BACE-2, which in turn led to the descriptor BACE-1 for the major β-secretase in AβPP processing. BACE-2 has 68% sequence homology to BACE-1, but differs in cellular and tissue localization, and acceptable substrates, and does not contribute to Aβ production.

BACE-1 cleaves AβPP at the expected sites on its extracellular domain at the start of Aβ, as well as a β' site 11 residues C-terminal to the start of Aβ. Interestingly, the AβPP670NL mutation immediately N-terminal to D at position 1 of Aβ is a more efficient substrate for BACE1 and generates higher levels of C terminal Aβ fragments and Aβ [59, 61, 62]. Moreover, knockout mouse studies have demonstrated that wild type and Swedish mutant AβPP670NL constructs require BACE-1 for Aβ production [63], and that BACE-1 knockout is compatible with survival, although there has been some suggestion that the knockout construct was not complete across both neurons and glia.

BACE-1 seems to accept a wide variety of substrates, and prefers acidic or polar residues in contrast to other aspartyl proteases, suggesting it is more like cathepsin D than renin in terms of substrate specificity [64]. BACE-1 cleaves at Asp at position 1 and Glu at position 11 as noted. Other fragments generated by cleavage at Val-3 and Ile-6 are produced by other as yet unidentified pathways. General rules for cleavage of BACE-1, based on amino acid sequence, have been suggested, whereas the requirements on the N-terminal side are more stringent than the C terminal side [55]. Various synthetic peptides have demonstrated differential binding affinities, suggesting a general property that longer peptide substrates are more effective, possibly because of a catalytic pocket for BACE-1-substrate interaction. Additionally, replacement of the natural cleavage site of AβPP with ISYEV leads to increases in the levels of the BACE-1 generated C terminal fragment, and Aβ, with a concomitant decrease in the α-secretase generated C terminal fragment [65].

BACE-1 is a type-I integral membrane glycoprotein with a 21-residue cleavable signal sequence, a large ectodomain of about 434 amino acides, a single transmembrane domain of about 22 amino acids, and a short cytoplasmic tail of 24 residues (Figure 2.7). A signal for intracellular transport motif in the C-terminal region is the acid cluster dileucine (ACDL) sequence, which facilitates intracellular protein trafficking [66, 67]. BACE-1 is a compact globular protein with two domains; the residues responsible for catalytic activity are encoded within the ectodomain. When comparing the structures of other mammalian aspartyl proteases, BACE-1 seems to have an extra loop, which could facilitate the addition of more subsites and increase the size of the target recognition site.

Post-translational modifications of BACE-1 include phosphorylation of a serine in the cytoplasmic domain [68], palmitoylation of three cysteines in the transmembrane and cytoplasmic domain, sulfation of the N-linked oligosaccharides [69], and glycosylation at four sites in the catalytic domain [70]. Three of these sites are modified in the endoplasmic reticulum and subsequently processed in the Golgi [70–72]. The significance of these four glocylation sites as it relates to catalytic activity and differential substrate specificity is of some interest in Aβ processing. Several studies have shown that cholesterol increases BACE-1 cleavage, although the mechanism is unclear [73, 74]. BACE-1 seems to be tissue specific, with preferential expression in neurons and pancreas. The broad physiological role for BACE-1 is nevertheless unresolved. BACE-1 appears to have a role in axonal growth, synaptic plasticity, and myelin production. As such, there is an implied role in cognition, albeit oblique.

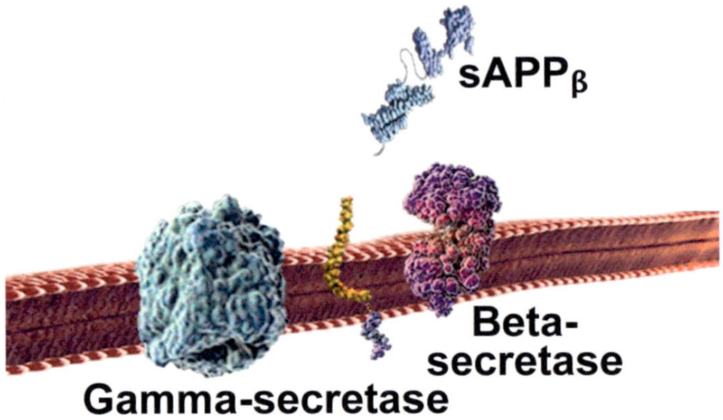

FIGURE 2.7: Three dimension schematic of the three membrane proteins, AβPP, β-secretase, and γ-secretase, necessary to generate Aβ peptides, is depicted.

Being centrally involved in the amyloid cascade concept as a rate-limiting factor, BACE-1 is attractive for therapeutically targeting Aβ. Preclinical studies have not surprisingly demonstrated efficacy in ameliorating Aβ and improving behavioral outcomes in transgenic mouse models. Unfortunately, a phase 2 clinical trial looking at the BACE inhibitor LY2886721 was halted due to liver abnormalities that showed up in four out of 45 patients during routine testing (http://newsroom.lilly.com/releasedetail.cfm?releaseid=771353).

2.4.2 Γ-SECRETASE

The complexity of the molecular pathology of AD is perhaps best illustrated by a discussion of γ-secretase, which is exceedingly complex and incompletely understood. γ-secretase activity was inferred by cell biology experiments, i.e., the generation of both 83 (C83, α-cleaved) and 99 (C99, β-cleaved) C-terminal AβPP fragments in addition to Aβ and the P3 fragment (see below), indicating an intramembrane cleavage of AβPP in addition to α- and β-secretase. Thus, C83 and C99 are substrates for a third enzyme, γ-secretase, at the cytoplasmic edge of the transmembrane domain (ε-site). The resulting C-terminal fragment (produced in the process of generating Aβ or P3), has received comparatively little attention, but translocation to the nucleus and interaction with transcription factors has been suggested [75–82]. The γ-secretase generating C-terminal fragment has also been shown to activate Fe65 at the cell surface, with secondary nuclear translocation and transcriptional activation [83].

The first evidence for a specific protein constituent of the enzyme complex was the finding that presenilin 1 (PS1), was required for γ-secretase activity [84]; this had in fact been predicted based on the existence of PS1-linked Familial AD. PS1 knockout constructs demonstrated a marked reduction in Aβ, and a concomitant increased C83 and C99. It is now generally accepted that PS1 is part of the catalytic domain of the γ-secretase complex, although some evidence against the simple conclusion is worth noting, such as the subcellular location of PS (primarily ER and early Golgi [85]) versus γ-secretase activity (cell surface as well as ER and Golgi [86–91]), and the apparent selectivity of the isocoumarin-type inhibitors that block the γ-secretase cleavage of AβPP but not Notch [92]. In either case, PS alone is not sufficient for protease activity. γ-secretase is said to be "promiscuous" with respect to AβPP cleavage, generating Aβ peptides ranging from 37 to 43 amino acids [93, 94].

RT-PCR analyses have demonstrated that PS1 and PS2 (gene on chromosome 1 linked to familial early onset AD) are expressed in most adult tissues and brain regions, with some evidence of differential regulation during development. PS1 expression overlaps with proteins BiP and calnexin [85, 95, 96], indicating that it principally resides within the Golgi during normal cellular metabolism. On the other hand, knockout experiments of PS2 have demonstrated little effect on AβPP metabolism and phenotypic development of transgenic animals, in contrast to PS1 knockout mice which have retarded embryonic growth and die shortly before or immediately after birth [97]. Combined PS1, PS2 knockout is an embryonic lethal at day 9.5. This suggests that PS1 is sufficient to compensate for lack of PS2, but the reverse is not true.

Limited structural data for γ-secretase is available, but it appears that γ-secretase is a diverse complex comprised of four essential subunits (Figure 2.8). Their precise interactions are technically challenging to study. The γ-secretase complex is comprised of four domains—APH-1, Nicastrin, Presenilin, and PEN-2—most likely in 1:1:1:1 stoichiometry [98]. PS again harbors the proteolytically active site, required for the putative aspartyl protease activity (Figure 2.9). Hydropathy plots have identified 10 hydrophobic regions, suggesting that PS contains seven to 10 transmembrane domains and is therefore an integral membrane protein [97]. PS1 and PS2 are both phosphorylated at serine residues although the significance of this modification is unknown. Nicastrin may function as a substrate receptor, although conflicting evidence exists. PEN-2 is thought to be required for PS stabilization within the catalytic domain. The function of APH-1 is unclear [98].

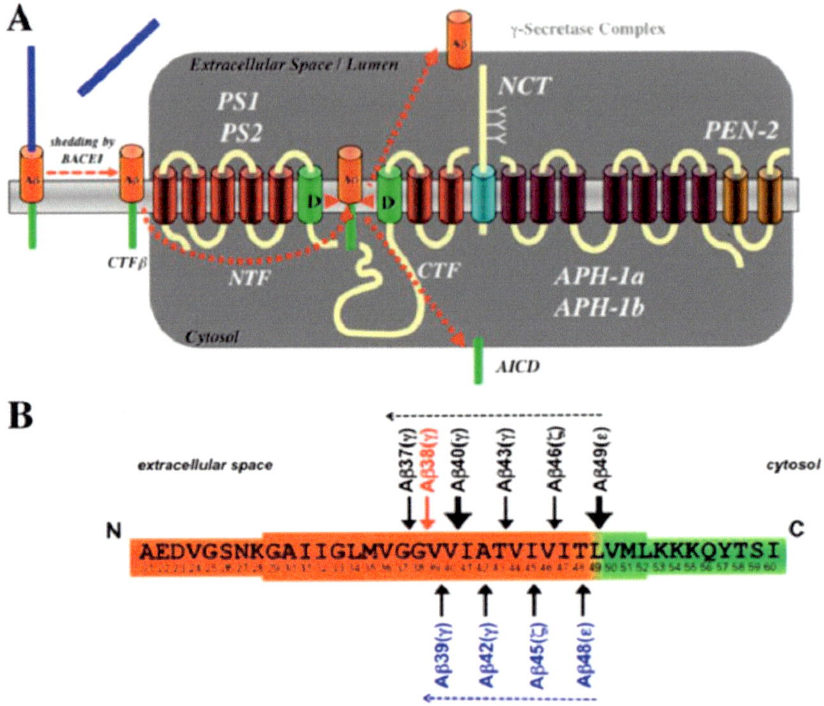

FIGURE 2.8: Figure 2.8A is a schematic representation of AβPP processing by β- and γ-secretases. Figure 2.8B shows multiple intramembrane cleavages are mediated by γ-secretase. The known cleavage sites and the resulting processing products are indicated. Major cleavage sites in the AβPP transmembrane domain are indicated by large arrows. The Aβ domain is depicted in orange, and the AβPP intracellular C-terminal domain (AICD) in green. The transmembrane domain is enlarged. Dashed arrows indicate the potential direction of the cleavages. NTF = N-terminal fragment.

The normal cellular function of γ-secretase is complicated by the limited overall structural data, and a multitude of potential functions of individual subunits, so not surprisingly bewildering arrays of cellular activity are plausible. Much of the functional data relates to the PS component, given its role as the putative catalytic site of the γ-secretase complex. Accepted roles include regulation of β-catenin and wnt-signaling, trafficking and degradation of membrane proteins, and substrate cleavage including AβPP [97]. PS, particularly PS2, has also been implicated in apoptosis and calcium signaling [99–102].

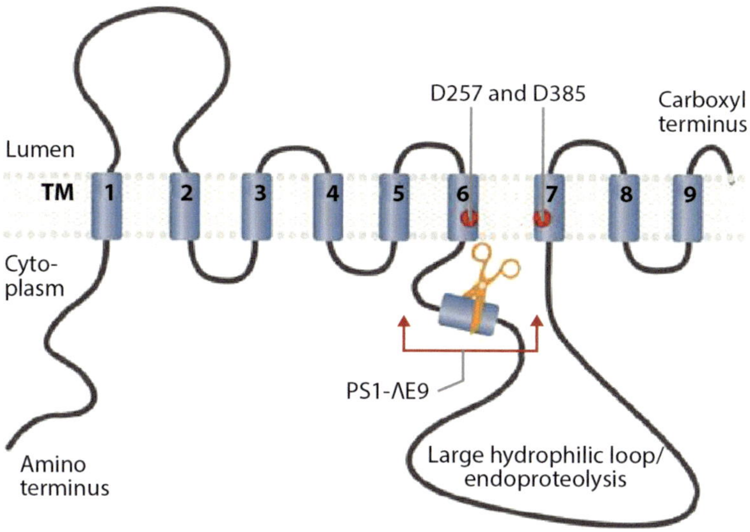

FIGURE 2.9: A schematic representation of presenilin, the catalytic site of the γ-secretase complex, is shown. Two aspartates (D257, D385) are required for endoproteolysis necessary to generate the functional complex of N- and C-terminal portions required for γ-secretase activity. Much about the γ-secretase complex and its role in health and disease is unknown, although involvement in Notch signaling indicates a highly conserved function (see text).

A broadly conserved role of PS in γ-secretase function was suggested by cloning of the presenilin ortholog in *C. elegans* termed Sel-12, found to be necessary for LIN-12/Notch signaling, a signaling cascade necessary for development of nematode vulva and other tissues [97, 103]. Notch is a single pass transmembrane receptor, originally discovered in *Drosophila*, where loss of function mutations produced a "notched" wing. It is thought to mediate cell–cell signaling which specifies cell fate within equivalence groups, indicating again an important developmental role.

Notch is activated by a proteolytic cascade with remarkable parallels with AβPP metabolism [97, 98, 103–105]. Briefly, Notch is constitutively cleaved by furin at cleavage site 1 during transport through the secretory pathway, which forms transmembrane intracellular Notch. With ligand binding, furin cleaved Notch undergoes a second cleavage at site 2. The ligand-bound extracellular domain is endocytosed, while the Notch extracellular truncation fragment remains within the plasma membrane. NEXT is the substrate for cleavage at site 3, which releases the Notch intracellular domain fragment from the membrane, which in turn allows nuclear translocation and transcriptional activation. NEXT is also cleaved at site 4, in the middle of the transmembrane domain to form the Nβ domain, similar to the p3 and Aβ peptides produced from cleavage of AβPP C83 and C99, respectively. The recognition that γ-secretase cleaves Notch suggests a role of protease cleavage in AβPP processing, and likewise that AβPP may act as a cell surface receptor.

In addition to Notch and AβPP, substrates for γ-secretase include epithelial cadherin (E-cadherin), ERbB-4, CD44—a surface receptor mediating cell adhesion, and Notch ligands Delta and Jagged. Finally, the N-terminal catalytically active site of PS is embedded in a conserved YD motif, whereas C-terminal active site domain contains an equally conserved GXGD-type aspartyl protease. Other GXGD-type aspartyl protease identified besides the γ-secretase/PS complex include procaryotic type 4 prepilin peptidases, and signal peptide peptidase, as well as the signal peptide peptidase-like proteases [98].

In short, γ-secretase cleavage is one small facet of prepilin peptidases, and SPP metabolism, and yet is exceedingly complex. Even a casual review breaches numerous biologically critical cellular processes, including growth and development, signal transduction by a variety of mechanisms, apoptosis, membrane turnover, and proteolysis. This only adds to the complexity of Aβ metabolism, indicates a multitude of potential roles in both health and disease, and serves as a reminder that our understanding of these and related processes is in its infancy.

2.4.3 A-SECRETASE

α-secretases are members of the ADAM ("a disintegrin and metalloprotease domain") family, expressed on cell surfaces and anchored to the plasma membrane [54]. Several such proteins, notably ADAM10, have been identified as possessing α-secretase activity. As noted above, prepilin peptidases, and AβPP processing by α-secretase results in C83, which therefore precludes production of full length Aβ peptide with subsequent γ-secretase cleavage, and is suggested to be both neuroprotective [106], and deficient in AD [107, 108]. The C83 fragment is nevertheless a substrate for γ-secretase, and leads to the production of an N terminal truncated fragment P3 by cleaving between residues 16 and 17 of Aβ, which paradoxically leaves behind a the amyloidogenic sequence of the Aβ molecule, and cleaves off the metal binding site. Likewise, although the α-secretase pathway is traditionally considered "non-amyloidogenic," and enhancing α-secretase activity has been shown experimentally to reduce Aβ production [109–111], the P3 fragment has been suggested as a model for oligomer formation and Aβ-mediated cytotoxicity [112, 113]. Here again Aβ metabolism is implicated as both beneficial and harmful, depending on the experimental construct.

2.5 SUMMARY OF ABPP PROCESSING

In summary, fully processed Aβ ranges from 37 to 43 amino acids, and is produced physiologically from processing of AβPP, a type-I transmembrane protein with an extracellular N-terminus and a cytosologic C-terminus. Processing of AβPP involves a complex interplay with three memebrane bound so-called secretases, α-secretase, β-secretase, and γ-secretase. α-secretase is in the ADAM family expressed on the cell surface and anchored to the plasma membrane. β-secretase, now called β-site AβPP cleavage enzyme-1, or BACE-1, is a membrane bound aspartyl protease with its active site in the extracellular space/endocytic lumen, and γ-secretase is an incompletely understood multiple protein complex with a catalytic site that involves presenilins, chromosome 14, and chromosome 1 proteins bearing pathogenic mutations that predispose to familial early onset dementia. β-secretase cleavage yields a 99 amino acid C terminal fragment, which is a substrate for subsequent γ-secretase cleavage, and which together yield the full length Aβ peptide, varying from 37 to 43 amino acids owning to promiscuity of the γ-secretase catalytic domain, which presumably PS (PS1 and/or PS2). Cleavage by β-secretase and γ-secretase is commonly referred to as the amyloidogenic pathway as it generates Aβ. Experimental studies suggest that the 42 amino acid Aβ species (Aβ40) has a tendency to deposit in neuritic plaques, has more neurotoxic features *in vitro* compared to the more common 40 amino acid Aβ species (Aβ 40), and is generally over-represented in familial AD when expressed as a ratio of Aβ42/Aβ40. Aβ42 is thus often referred to as the "culprit" or pathogenic Aβ species according to amyloid cascade dogma. In contrast, cleavage by α-secretase generates an 83 amino acid C terminal AβPP fragment, which is also a substrate for γ-secretase and which, when cleaved by both α-secretase and γ-secretase, generates the so-called P3 fragment, which is in essence truncated Aβ devoid of its metal binding region but retaining the amyloidogenic region. The P3 fragment is said to be irrelevant with respect to pathology, although some studies have raised the possibility that the P3 fragment may mediate cellularity cytotoxicity. All of the above also ignores the alternative viewpoint, that Aβ synthesis is an evolutionarily conserved, adaptive response.

Cellular trafficking studies of AβPP indicate that AβPP undergoes N- and O-linked glycosylation, tyrosine sulfation, and phosphorylation (cytoplasmic) between the ER and plasma membrane. However, only about 10% of AβPP is at the cell surface, while the bulk of AβPP localizes to the golgi and trans-golgi network. AβPP that is not secreted is rapidly internalized, recycled to the plasma membrane, or degraded via a highly regulated process. Despite the intense interest in AβPP processing, regulatory factors affecting trafficking of AβPP and secretases in the human brain, and their relationship, if any, to disease, are poorly understood.

2.6 IMPLICATIONS OF FAMILIAL AD IN THE MOLECULAR PATHOLOGY

AβPP processing necessarily invites a discussion of familial AD, as it is the existence of familial AD that serves as the foundation for the present belief system as regards the molecular pathogenesis of AD (Table 2.2). The vast majority of kindreds affected by familial early onset AD demonstrate pathogenic mutations involving AβPP, PS1, and PS2. According to the Alzheimer's Disease and

Frontotemporal Dementia mutation data base, 33 AβPP mutations are described in 90 families, 185 PS1 mutations are described in 405 families, and 13 PS2 mutations are described in 22 families (http://www.molgen.ua.ac.be/ADMutations/). It is interesting that PS1 mutations comprise about 80% of those causes of familial disease, and emphasizes the role of the γ-secretase complex in AβPP metabolism. Classical concepts suggest that PS1 mutations enhance γ-secretase activity, thereby generating increased Aβ, although some studies suggest an overall decrease in Aβ production [114], and that the increased Aβ42:Aβ40 ratio commonly accepted as central to disease in PS1 mutation cases, is actually due to a decrease in Aβ40 [115] rather than increased Aβ42. It might also be kept in mind that if the total number of families that have been identified, slightly more than 500 worldwide, are at all representative of the total, familial disease pales in comparison to sporadic disease [11], which is said to affect more than 5 million individuals in the United States alone, criticisms of overdiagnosis notwithstanding (http://www.theguardian.com/society/2013/sep/10/dementia-over-diagnosis).

TABLE 2.2: Familial Alzheimer's Disease (http://www.molgen.ua.ac.be/ADMutations)

Gene	# of Mutations	# of Families
APP	33	90
PSEN1	185	405
PSEN2	13	22

The mechanisms by which mutation causes disease are diverse and complex. Indeed, a recently identified APP "mutation," A673T, showed some statistical evidence for preservation of cognitive function associated with the mutation [116]. The nature of the disease in PS1 mutation cases (early onset, severe pathology) suggest a toxic gain of function, although this is far from clear and some have suggested a loss of function in PS1 mutation, with Aβ accumulating simply because of altered processing and a change in steady state in favor of Aβ, as opposed to overexpression and increased production *per se* [114, 117]. Although comprising only about 15% of the familial cases, AβPP mutation is perhaps easier to understand on a mechanistic level, yet even in the case of AβPP mutation, the molecular pathology is complex. For example, in Swedish mutation cases there is an increase in total Aβ because mutation in the amino Aβ terminus results in a more efficient substrate for BACE1 cleavage [63, 118]. Mutation of the C terminus of Aβ (e.g., Austrian, Iranian, French, German, London, Florida mutations) are said to cause disease by favoring overproduction of the putative neurotoxic species, Aβ42. Mutations in the mid Aβ region (e.g., Dutch, Arctic) are said to alter the primary structure of Aβ resulting in an enhanced propensity toward aggregation. The Flemish mutation is suggested to diminish the activity of an AβPP domain that normally exerts an inhibitory influence on the γ-secretase complex [54]. Each of these mechanisms can just as easily be reasoned in the opposite direction with an abundance of evidence, and is a reminder that genetics involves significance rather than causality. AβPP metabolism and Aβ formation is clearly a central feature of AD and nomrla aging, but causality is not demonstrated.

The empirical data may give one pause as well. PS1 mutation cases are marked by both clinical and pathological heterogeneity. Clinically, onset before age 30 has been described in numerous kindreds [119]. There may be a long prodromal phase with subtle deficits in some cognitive domains and not others, and in a pattern and temporal progression not encountered in sporadic AD. Seizure and myoclonus are invariable in some kindreds, and absent in others. Dystonia, parkinsonism, and marked orthostatic hypotension, are variably described. Behavioral and psychiatric symptoms more in line with frontotemporal dementia phenotype are seen in a number of kindreds [120]. In G184V PS1 mutation subjects, neuropathological expression was that of Pick disease without AD plaques [121]. Early aphasia is present in some kindreds, visual agnosia, and cerebellar ataxia are variably present depending on the kindred. Spastic paraparesis may be prominent, particularly among exon 9 mutations [38, 122]. In terms of pathology, NFT formation may be sparse or prodigious, depending on the mutation. Cotton wool plaques which lack an amyloid core and neuritic changes are often the predominant plaque form, a feature essentially never encountered in sporadic AD to any significant degree [38]. Cerebellar pathology may be particularly severe and accompanied by neuritic pathology, a finding not seen in sporadic AD [123]. Amyloid angiopathy may be extreme and lead to intracerebral hemorrhage as a cause of death, or may be absent [54, 124]. Lewy body pathology is frequent in PSEN cases [125]. It is also interesting to note that APP mutation kindreds were first identified not as familial AD, but familial cerebral hemorrhage with amyloidosis. AβPP692 (Flemish) mutation subjects have severe cerebral amyloid angiopathy, frequent hemorrhage, abundant cored amyloid plaques in the cerebellum, and abundant neurofibrillary pathology [126]. In contrast, AβPP693 (Dutch) subjects have limited to absent neurofibrillary pathology, plaque pathology that is typically of the diffuse type, in addition to characteristic intracerebral hemorrhage.

Familial late-onset AD is often attributed to ApoE genotype, since ApoE ε4 alleles confer increased risk for AD, although it should be noted that ApoE alleles are polymorphic rather than mutated, so strictly speaking are not indicative of "familial" disease. ApoE co-localizes with Aβ in plaque pathology, and is suggested to promote fibrillogenesis by experimental studies [127]. The relationship between ApoE and neuropathology, however, is complex [128]. In one study of two AD brains homozygous ε4 genotype, there was a noteworthy lack of the defining feature of sporadic AD pathology, the neuritic plaque [129].

None of the clinical and neuropathological heterogeneity in familial AD kindreds is particularly surprising, and in some respects is expected. It does serve as a reminder, however, that pathogenic mutations are by definition aberrations. Given the complexity of AβPP metabolism and secretase processing in general, the extent of disruption of the molecular environment imposed by pathogenic mutation is probably only beginning to be understood. It might also be kept in mind that the amyloid cascade concept is based purely on genetic aberration [32]. W hereas disease modeling and preclinical studies are based on pathogenic mutation, i.e., familial AD, all therapeutic targeting to date has been directed at sporadic AD. Whether this explains, at least in part, the therapeutic failures, may be answered by recent trials involving familial AD.

CHAPTER 3

Neurofibrillary Degeneration

3.1 PATHOLOGY

The neurofibrillary tangle is typically mentioned alongside the plaque as the second hallmark lesion of AD, although it may be useful at the outset to use the more encompassing term, "neurofibrillary degeneration" in reference to accumulation of phosphorylated tau *per se* rather than subcellular compartment (i.e., neurofibrillary tangle is accumulation of perikaryal phosphorylated tau; neuropil thread is axonal or dendritic accumulation of phosphorylated tau; dystrophic neurites are accumulation of phosphorylated tau in swollen or "dystrophic" dendritic or axonal processes in the vicinity of plaques) (Figure 3.1). Phospho-tau accumulation within the cytoplasm of macroglia (e.g., astrocytes, oligodendrocytes) is also increasingly recognized with age [130], in various neurodegenerative conditions, and in so-called chronic traumatic encephalopathy [131] [Table 3.1].

The original description of the neurofibrillary tangle is attributable to Alzheimer [1], while dystrophic neurites were probably originally described by Oskar Fischer as noted above [18]. Neurofibrillary pathology and in particular neurofibrillary tangles are intensely argyrophilic using the Bielschowsky silver technique, and readily demonstrated using immunohistochemistry to phosphorylated tau. Routine dyes such hematoxylin and eosin rather faintly stain neurofibrillary tangles and a subset of dystrophic neurites, and generally do not highlight neuropil threads at all.

Like the plaque, neurofibrillary degeneration is a basic reaction of the central nervous system and is not specific for any clinical condition other than the passage of time. The earliest accumulations of phosphorylated tau epitopes as defined by large scale immunohistochemistry have even been described in youth [130] and a long list of conditions typified by at least focal neurofibrillary degeneration therefore exists [132]. Nevertheless, clinicians and neuropathologists are increasingly invoking the term "tauopathy" for those conditions in which phospho-tau accumulation is the predominant pathological findings. This is sometimes used in contrast to "synucleinopathy" for those conditions in which alpha-synuclein accumulates (e.g., Parkinson disease, Lewy body dementia, multiple system atrophy). While reasonable as a descriptive term, the use of the "opathy" suffix also carries the unfortunate appeal that the protein in question, or aberrant metabolism of that protein, is etiological. This in turn lends itself to a competing, but equally reductionist, protein cascade to explain neurodegeneration, and the continuing basic transposition of cause and effect. The neurobiologist would again be well served to keep in mind that life itself is a progressive tauopathy.

Phospho-tau accumulation may therefore be viewed as a reactive phenomenon, in order to avoid the pitfall of burying oneself in the gray zone between pathology and physiology [133].

TABLE 3.1: Diseases with tau neuropathology (modified from Wolfe, 2009) [141]
Frontotemporal dementia and parkinsonism linked to chromosome 17 (FTDP-17)
Alzheimer's Disease
Aging
Progressive supranuclear palsy
Pick's disease
Argyrophilic grain dementia
Corticobasal degeneration
Progressive subcortical gliosis
Amyotrophic lateral sclerosis/parkinsonism-dementia complex
Diffuse neurofibrillary tangles with calcification
Dementia pugilistica (Chronic traumatic encephalopathy)
Tangle-only dementia
Down syndrome
Gerstmann-Straussler-Scheinker disease
Hallervorden-Spatz disease
Creutzfeldt-Jakob disease
Multiple system atrophy
Niemann-Pick disease type C
Prion protein cerebral amyloid angiopathy
Subacute sclerosing panencephalitis
Myotonic dystrophy
Non-guanamian motor neuron disease with neurofibrillary tangles
Postencephalitic parkinsonism
Meningioangiomatosis
Tuberous Sclerosis

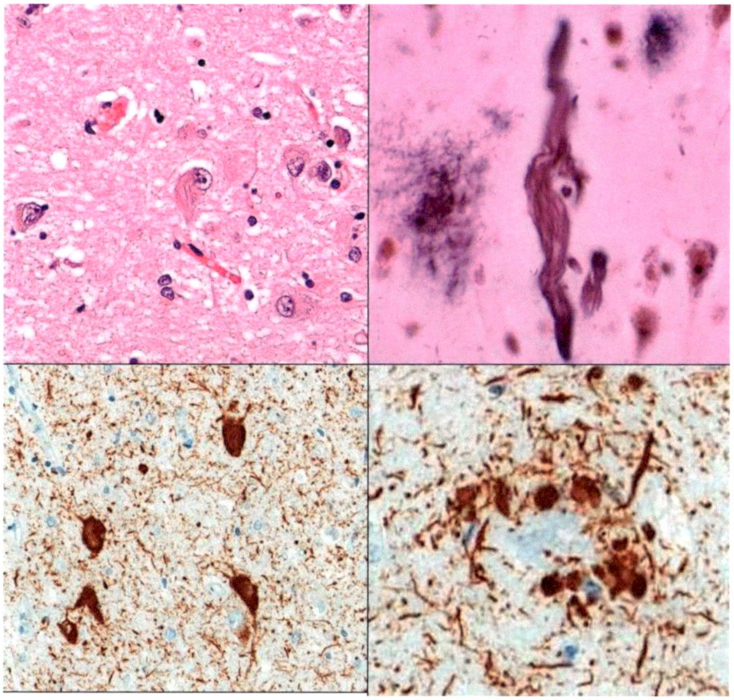

FIGURE 3.1: Neurofibrillary degeneration is generally comprised of neurofibrillary tangles, neuropil threads, and dystrophic neurites, although there are many other morphological expressions of tau pathology. Figure 3.1A shows a neurofibrillary tangle (NFT) on a routine hematoxylin and eosin preparation. NFTs stain faintly with routine dyes, which may be why they were unidentified until the advent of Bielschowsky silver staining (Figure 3.1B is a silver-positive neurofibrillary tangle). AT8 immunohistochemistry (C and D) is another sensitive indicator of hyperphosphorylated tau in tissues. Figure 3.1C shows several neurofibrillary tangles as well as abundant neuropil threads. Figure 3.1D shows dystrophic neurites within a neuritic plaque, in addition to an abundance of neuropil threads.

Little progress was made into the constituents of the NFT over numerous decades following its description. This can be attributed in large part to slow technological advances. Prior to the 1980s, understanding of the NFT was purely morphological. Divry (1934) made the erroneous observation that they were largely extracellular because they were Congo red positive and showed green birefringence with plane polarization [134]. This was successfully refuted three decades later by the ultrastructural description of NFT by Kidd in 1963 [135]. In this brief but seminal paper, Kidd described NFT as being comprised of paired helical filaments, the individual filaments 100 angstroms in thickness, the pair coming to regular constrictions of 150 angstroms, and with the paired helices completing a turn lengthwise every 1600 angstroms when viewed parallel to the plane of section (Figure 3.2). Kidd commented that "The tendency of these pathological filaments to stain with Congo red suggests a similarity to amyloid, but the latter is known to be extracellular, and these filaments are intracellular." Prior to these observations, there was some debate as to whether the protein constituents of NFT were the same as the plaque. This paper highlighted a clear divergence from that suggestion.

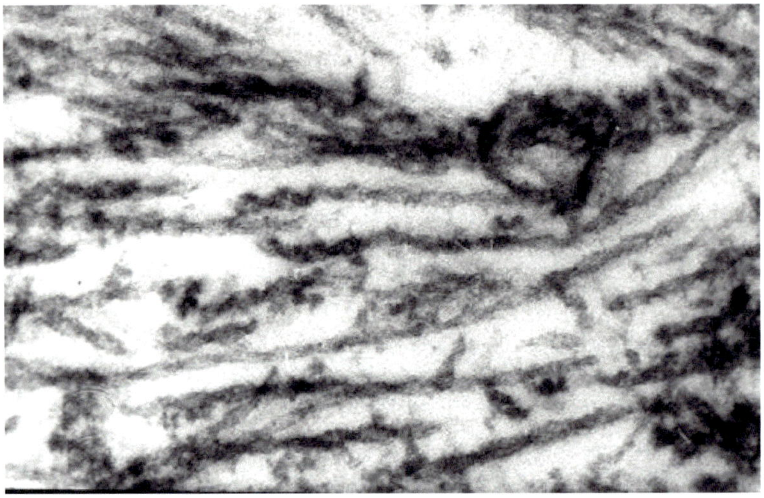

FIGURE 3.2: Kidd in 1963 was the first to demonstrate the ultrastructural characteristics of neurofibrillary degeneration, which consisted of intracellular of paired helical filaments, settling the controversy about whether they were intracellular and extracellular, and casting doubt on whether they were comprised of the same material as amyloid plaques. The filaments individually measure about 10 nm, and complete one turn of the helix every 160 nm [135].

3.2 PURIFICATION OF TAU

The most substantial advance in the molecular biology of the NFT was made by Inge Grudke-Iqbal and colleagues in the mid-1980s, around the same time than Aβ was being purified and sequenced. Bulk isolation and purification initially yielded polypeptides that failed to migrate on SDS-PAGE with a number of known cytoskeletal elements, including neurofilament, tubulin, actin, and myosin [136]. Antibodies raised against PHF absorbed with purified PHF protein but failed to absorb with identically prepared neurofilament protein [137], a long-suspected constituent of PHF. Eventually, the lately characterized tau protein was purified from bovine brain microtubules by five different techniques [138]. Each purified preparation reacted to anti-sera to PHF, and in a follow up study, monoclonal antibodies to the low molecular weight microtubule-associated protein tau labeled

NFT and neurites, with enhanced staining following dephosphorylation, confirming that the major protein component of PHF was phosphorylated tau protein [139].

3.3 TAU BIOLOGY

The gene for the microtubule associated protein tau (MAPT) is located on 17q21 and contains 16 exons. Exons 1, 4, 5, 7, 9, 11, and 12 are constitutive exons (Figure 3.3). Exons 2, 3, and 10 are alternatively spliced, resulting in differential expression in the adult brain [132, 140, 141]. Tau belongs to the group of microtubule-associated proteins as noted, which demonstrate heat resistance and limited susceptibility to acid hydrolysis. These properties are most likely the result of limited secondary structure with significant lack of folding in the native state, which explains why the structure of tau is better demonstrated with nuclear magnetic resonance spectroscopy over x-ray crystallography.

Six tau isoforms differ according to alternative splicing of exons 2, 3, and 10 [141]. Exons 2 and 3 each code for 29 amino acids. Inclusion of exon 2 is coupled to exon 3 but not *vice versa.* Tau isoforms could therefore be designated 2N (includes both exons 2 and 3), 1N (exon 3 only), and 0N (includes neither exon 2 nor exon 3). Exon 10 encodes 31 or 32 amino acids and the second of four possible microtubule binding domains. Alternative splicing of exon 10 may therefore result in three repeats (3R) when exon 10 is not included, and four repeats (4R) when exon 10 is included. The six isoforms are therefore possible in this scenario: three 3R tau (contain 0N, 1N, and 2N depending on exon 2 and exon 3 splicing, and three 4R tau isoforms, again 0N, 1N, and 2N depending on exon 2 and exon 3 splicing. Each of these isoforms are differentially expressed during development, with 3R tau with no inserts expressed in the fetus, and one or two N-terminal inserts with 4R tau expressed during adulthood. Moreover, the relative abundances of 3R and 4R tau are empirical markers of disease subtype, and implicated as pathogenic in the so-called tauopathies. Pick disease, for example, contains predominantly 3R tau. Progressive supranuclear palsy and corticobasal degeneration contain predominantly 4R tau. AD and chronic traumatic encephalopathy contain a mixture of 3R and 4R, while argyrophilic grain disease, a putative entity with variable clinical correlates, appears to be a 4R tauopathy. These differences have been explained in part by intronic mutations affecting exon 10 splicing, without affecting primary structure. Not surprisingly, differential processing of tau is implicated in the pathogenesis of the tauopathies.

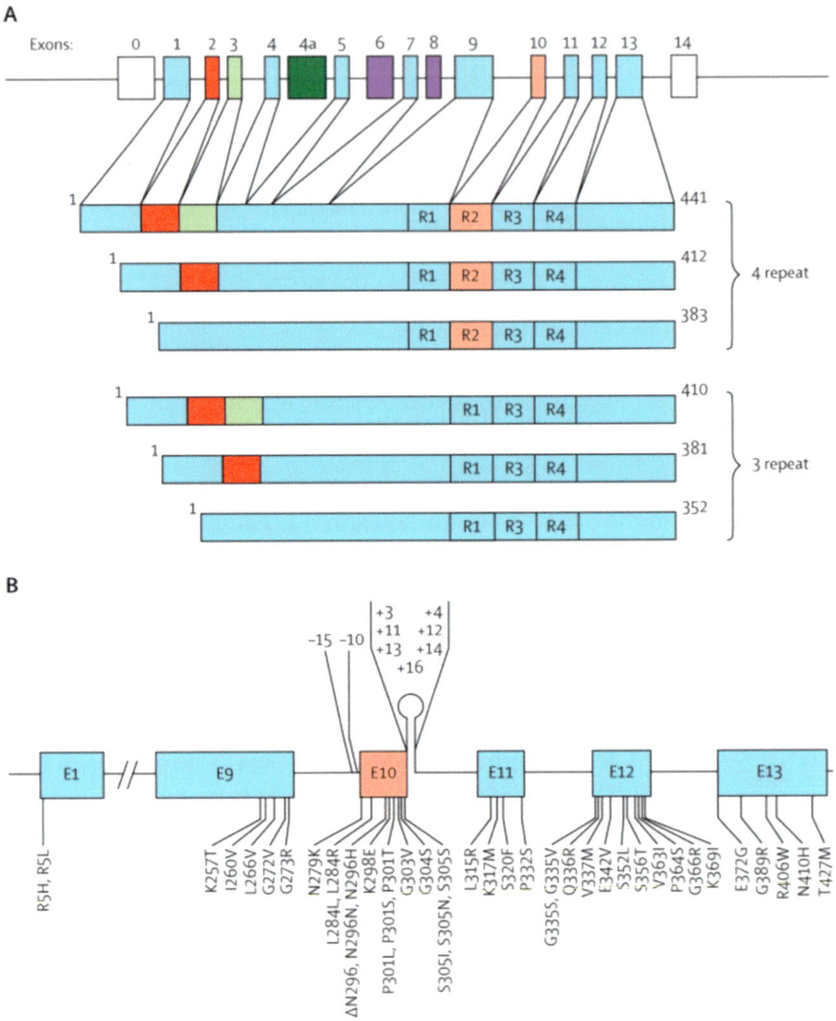

FIGURE 3.3 [202]: Tau protein gene (MAPT, Figure 3.3A) and the six tau isoforms expressed in an adult human brain are depicted. MAPT consists of 16 exons (E). Alternative mRNA splicing of E2 (red), E3 (light green), and E10 (orange) gives rise to the six tau isoforms (amino acids 352–441). The constitutively spliced exons (E1, E4, E5, E7, E9, E11, E12, and E13) are shown in blue. E0, which is part of the promoter, and E14 are non-coding (white). E6 and E8 (violet) are not transcribed in human brain. E4a (dark green) is expressed only in the peripheral nervous system. The repeats of tau (R1–R4) are shown, with three isoforms having four repeats each (4 repeat) and three isoforms having three repeats each (3 repeat). Each repeat is 31 or 32 aminoacids in length. Figure 3.3B shows utations in MAPT in cases of frontotemporal dementia and parkinsonism linked to chromosome 17 (FTDP-17T). 42 coding-region mutations in MAPT and nine intronic mutations flanking E10 are shown. Used with permission from Jucker and Walker [203].

The N-terminal region encoded by exons 2 and 3 give rise to the so-called projection domain as it projects of the surface of the microtubule and may interact with other cytoskeletal elements [140]. As such, the variable size of this domain may determine axon diameter. Long projection axons in the peripheral nervous system, for example, contain an additional N-terminal motif encoded on exon 4A resulting in a species called "big tau." Tau interacts with other cytoskeletal elements including actin and spectrin, which may in turn influence interaction with neurofilaments, restricting mobility and stabilization of the microtubule polymer, and possibly explaining why neurofilament domains are incorporated into neurofibrillary degneration [142]. The N terminal region further interacts with membrane elements of organelles including mitochondria and the plasma membrane, implying a role in organelle transport.

The repeat region of tau, encoded by exons 9 through 12, each coding for 18 residues that are highly conserved and imperfectly repeated, comprise the microtubule binding domain. The main function of tau appears to be its promotion of microtubule assembly at the expense of disassembly, a process that is more robust in the adult compared to the fetus. The specific subregion implicated as the most potent promoter of microtubule assembly is an inter-region between repeat 1 and repeat 2, and more specifically the peptide sequence KVQIINKK. This sequence is unique to adult tau and specifies as well 4R tau. Given these features and intimate association with microtubules, it is not surprising that tau protein is broadly implicated in cellular processes apart from neurodegeneration, including growth and development, cell division, cytoskeletal elements encompassing molecular and organelle trafficking via motor proteins and axonal transport, endocytic pathways, and membrane turnover.

The identification of tau within paired helical filaments of AD was accompanied by evidence of tau phosphorylation in disease, which has been studied extensively ever since. Phosphorylation of tau is now considered an important regulator of microtubule binding by tau and associated pleiotropic effects. A steady state level of tau phosphorylation is physiologic, while hyperphosphorylation effects disassembly and loss of function. The highest molecular weight form of tau possesses 80 potential serine/threonine phosphorylation sites, although phosphorylation specific monoclonal antibodies combined with mass spectrometry and sequencing indicate about 30 phosphorylation sites that can be occupied: Thr39, Ser46Pro, Thr50Pro, Thr69Pro, Thr153Pro, Thr175Pro, Thr181Pro, Ser198, Ser199Pro, Ser202Pro, Thr205Pro, Ser208, Ser210, Thr212Pro, Ser214, Thr217Pro, Thr-231Pro, Ser235Pro, Ser237, Ser241, Ser262, Ser285, Ser305, Ser324, Ser352, Ser356, Ser396Pro, Ser400, Thr403, Ser404Pro, Ser409, Ser412, Ser413, Ser416 and Ser422Pro. All of these sites are in the vicinity of, but still outside, the microtubule-binding domains, with the exception of Ser 262 (R1), Ser285 (R1–R2 inter-repeat), Ser305 (R2–R3 inter-repeat), Ser324 (R3), Ser352 (R4), and Ser356 (R4).

While phosphorylation of tau is the molecular correlate to one of two principle hallmark lesions in AD, it is imprecisely defined as "inappropriate" or "abnormal" phosphorylation [143].

Biochemical properties of phosphorylated tau are also loosely defined, and encompass altered molecular weight/electrophoretic mobility, conformational change included increased β-sheet content, detergent insolubility, increased overall phosphorylation, and non-physiologic or inappropriate phosphorylation of specific residues. Noteworthy from the pathogenesis perspective is that abnormally phosphorylated tau in AD neither binds microtubules nor promotes microtubule assembly. It may further prevent normal tau from binding microtubules, shifting the balance in favor of the cytosolic phase. Indeed, even in NFT affected neurons, as much as 40% of the phosphorylated tau is depolymerized and not a component of paired helical filaments [143]. Recovery of normal tau function with dephosphorylation was noted in a cellular model of tau phosphorylation [141].

The precise mechanism of tau phosphorylation is unknown, although perterbations in kinase-phosphatase are broadly implicated. Among kinases, glycogen synthase kinase-3β (GSK-3β) has received the most attention [143]. GSK-3β phosphorylates tau at 14 sites, with substantial overlap with AD tau phosphorylation. Transgenic animal studies using FTDP-17 triple transgene show reduction of pathology and tau phosphorylation with administration of lithium chloride, an inhibitor of GSK-3β. Changes in tau affinity for microtubules as a function of GSK-3β phosphorylation have been shown, as has GSK-3β-induced formation of NFT-like structures from synthetic tau. Among other kinases implicated in abnormal tau phosphorylation are cyclin-dependent kinase-5, cAMP-dependent protein kinase, and calcium/calmodulin-dependent kinase II. On the other hand, the opposite effect by phosphatases is both theoretical and empirically demonstrated for PP1, PP2A, PP2B, and PP2C, which dephosphorylated tau *in vitro*. PP2A activity has been shown to be reduced in the AD brain. Not surprisingly, the AD brain contains substantially more phosphorylated tau than cognitively intact aged individuals [143].

The attractiveness of dysfunctional tau metabolism as a primary or rate limiting factor in AD is substantiated by the involvement of tau in a plethora of critical metabolic activities within neurons as noted above. Neurofibrillary degeneration and phosphorylated tau accumulation, moreover, is more closely aligned with neurological signs, neuropathological stage, and clinical and pathological disease severity as compared to accumulations of Aβ [30, 130]. Hampering the perceived importance of phosphorylated tau, and perhaps unduly so, is disease phenotype in familial disease linked to tau gene mutation, much like AβPP-linked familial disease unduly influences the perception of the importance of Aβ [141]. To date, 44 MAPT mutations (frontotemporal dementia with parkinsonism linked to chromosome 17 (FTDP-17)) have been described in a total of 134 families, comprising a substantial percentage of familial dementia kindreds (http://www.molgen.ua.ac.be/ADMutations/). Disease phenotype, however, is more in line with frontotemporal dementia, with clinical signs often affecting behavior, language, and motor function. Other cases may resemble sporadic tauopathies including corticobasal degeneration, progressive supranuclear palsy, and Pick disease, but only uncommonly display an AD-like clinical phenotype, and in general are not accompanied by significant plaque pathology. Most of the mutations are missense mutations and tend to cluster in the C-terminal region or in an intronic segment near exon 10. C-terminal mutations adversely affect microtubule assembly and disrupt all tau isoforms, while exon 10 mutations only affect the three 4R isoforms, owing to the requirement of exon 10 to produce 4R tau. A number of tau mutation transgenic mice have been developed, of which the P301S model is probably the most widely utilized.

3.4 GRANULOVACUOLAR DEGENERATION

Granulovacuolar degeneration (GVD) was described in patients with senile dementia by Simchowitz in 1911 [144]. They have since been described in Pick disease, amyotrophic lateral sclerosis (ALS), tuberous sclerosis, Down syndrome, the dementia-ALS-parksinson complex of guam, and aging, and are generally not regarded as specific for AD [145–147]. They are nevertheless described in major texts as an accompaniment of AD and merit brief discussion. GVD is characterized morphologically by the presence of discrete 0.5–5 μm basophilic granules, each within a clear vacuole, in the perikaryal cytoplasm of pyramidal neurons (Figure 3.4). They are most apparent in the medial temporal lobe where they show a hierarchy of neuronal involvement, from subiculum, to CA-1, to CA-2 [148]. They also occur in pyramidal neurons of the neocortex and olfactory bulb [149]. The granules contain an electron dense core surrounded by a translucent matrix on ultrastructural analysis, and have been shown to express a number of epitopes, such as neurofilament protein, phospho-tau, ubiquitin, prolyl peptidyl isomerase 1, and, mitotic proteins TG-3, and MPM-2 [150–154]. Cellular function implicated in the histogenesis of GVD include the autophagic ubiquitin proteasome system, unfolded protein response, endosomal and lysosomal proteins, tau and amyloid-β processing events, and stress- and mitogen-activated protein induction [153, 155–158]. There seems to be a lack of correlation between GVD and neurofibrillary degeneration [159, 160], although other studies report an association between the two [148].

In a recent study, we found phosphorylated ribosomal protein S6 (pS6), a protein associated with the 40S ribosomal subunit in eukaryotes with a role in RNA storage, degradation, and re-entry into translation, immunolocalized to GVD [161]. pS6 levels were also higher in AD neurons and inversely related to apoptosis and NFT. Since pS6 is a specific marker for stress granules, which are high conserved markers of molecular triage process in situations of cellular stress (e.g., oxidative stress, ischemia) [162, 163], GVD may be a morphological marker of stress granules formation and environmental adaptation in humans. Although not specific for AD, GVD may be no less specific than Aβ plaques or NFT.

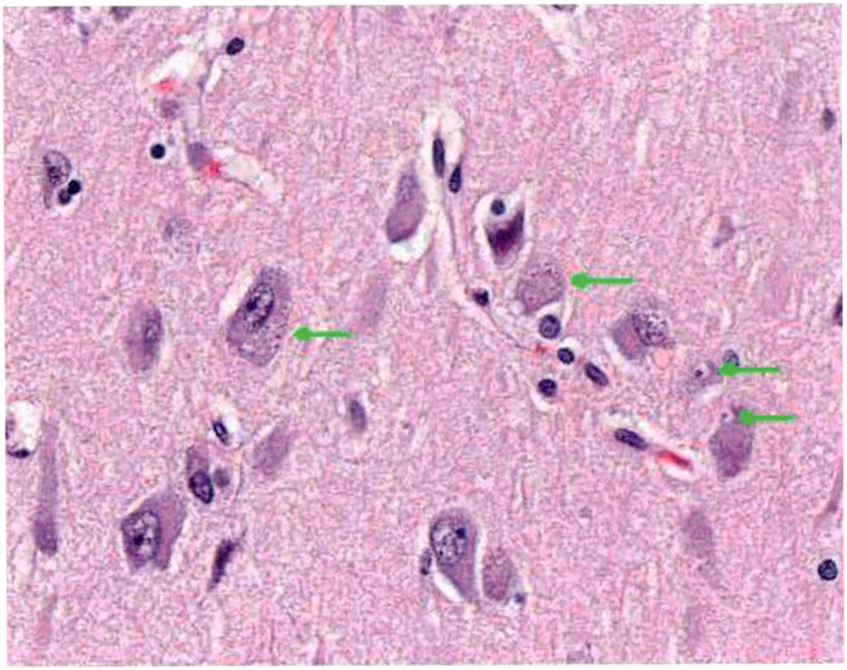

FIGURE 3.4: A high magnification section of hippocampal pyramidal neurons shows granulovacuolar degeneration (GVD) (arrows). GVD is seen with age and in a number of conditions as a probable morphological indicator of response to cellular stress.

CHAPTER 4
Complexities

4.1 REGIONAL DISTRIBUTION OF PLAQUES AND TANGLES

A linear protein construct with Aβ in an upstream position and phospho-tau in a downstream position is immediately apparent with even a casual glance at the various iterations of the amyloid cascade hypothesis. The complexity of the brain, however, may preclude such reductionist schema *in vivo*. Regional variation in Aβ and phospho-tau is a case in point. Aβ accumulation tends to accumulate first in the cerebral neocortex, but with otherwise little region specificity [164]. In a recent study, we showed accumulation of Aβ-positive diffuse plaques initially in prefrontal cortex of middle aged but cognitively intact apolipoprotein ε4 homozygoes (most of whom would have presumably gone on to develop late onset AD), with no discernible Aβ elsewhere (in preparation). In disease, Aβ accumulation is considered to progress from neocortex, to allocortex, to deep gray matter, to cerebellum as disease advances [30]. The reasons for this are obscure and nearly entirely uninvestigated when compared to basic neuroscience studies presuming AβPP as a neurotoxic starting point. There is further no evidence that the regional distribution of Aβ relates in any way to differences in regional or cellular APP transcription. Why some brain regions readily accumulate Aβ with age and disease, while other brain regions accumulate little to none, even with end-stage disease, is a complete mystery. Regional variation of Aβ pathology as of this writing is entirely unexplained.

In contrast to Aβ, the earliest accumulations of phospho-tau appear in the brainstem, followed by limbic structures, association cortices, and finally primary neocortical areas [130]. Moreover, phospho-tau generally appears in the brainstem prior to Aβ appearing in the neocortex. These simple data again defy the linear Aβ-phospho-tau construct from the standpoint of reality, or the human brain *in vivo*. Similarly, the mechanistic basis for the early accumulation phospho-tau in some populations (e.g., locus ceruleus) and the late or absent accumulation phospho-tau in others, (e.g., cerebellar Purkinje cells), even with end-stage disease, is non-existent. The empirical data nevertheless demonstrate convincingly that there is a spatial and temporal disconnect between the accumulations of Aβ and phospho-tau, and that each can and does accumulate in the absence of the other [130, 164, 165]. Aβ and phospho-tau tend to converge with disease, but then only with advanced to end-stage disease, and only above the tentorium for reasons that are obscure (Figure

4.1). So "although one might be tempted to do so, one cannot relate plaques to fibrillary change, and vice versa."

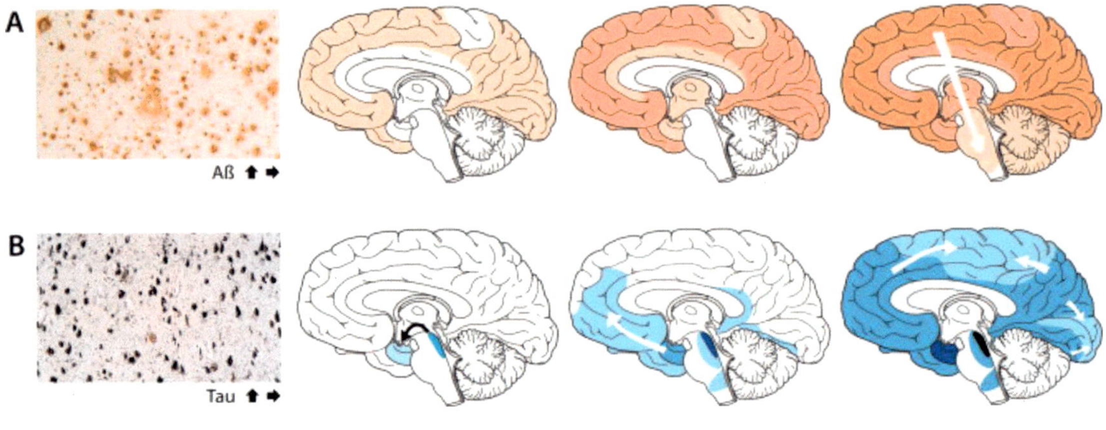

FIGURE 4.1: The accumulation of Aβ and phospho-tau in Alzheimer's Disease follows fundamentally different patterns, indicating a spatial and temporal disconnect between in aging and disease. Cross-sectional autopsy studies indicate that Aβ appears in the neocortex, followed by the allocortex, brainstem, and cerebellum. Phospho-tau (B) appears first in the brainstem, followed by transentorhinal area, limbic cortex, association cortex, and primary cortical areas. Modified and used with permission from Jucker and Mathias, 2011 [203].

4.2 OLIGOMERS

Although strictly speaking the so-called oligomer bears no relationship with pathology *in vivo*, some brief discussion on the oligomer as it relates to neuropathology is warranted. The identification of soluble Aβ species was noted first by Gambetti and colleagues in the 1990s, although at that time the focus of most laboratories was on insoluble Aβ and fibril toxicity as the mediator of disease in AD [166]. Problematic, however, was the capricious relationship between Aβ neuropathology and disease, its lack of specificity, and the frequent identification of abundant plaque pathology in cognitively intact elderly [128, 167–169]. Indeed, as mentioned above, the recognition of plaque pathology in non-demented individuals dates prior to Alzheimer's Disease of Auguste D. [170]. However, the new knowledge of AβPP metabolism, and the elaboration of the simple, if not pre-ordained, amyloid cascade concept, led to a massive proliferation of *in vitro* studies of Aβ, and biochemical properties that were not intuitively obvious, at least on a prospective basis.

Oligomers are basically defined as low-n mers of Aβ protein that remain in solution following high speed centrifugation [171]. The existence of such a transition state is predicted by the presence of a monomer of Aβ produced by β-secretease and γ-secretase cleavage on the one hand, and the plaque comprised of aggregated, fibillary Aβ on the other, i.e., an intermediary state between elaboration and nucleation [172]. By definition, such a transition state is an *in vitro* or at best *ex vivo* construct and as such difficult to define *in vivo* where they in fact may not exist due to differences in nucleation. So oligomers remain more a concept than a pathologic reality.

Even assuming the oligomer is pathophysiologically relevant, there is a staggering list of potential Aβ species, produced by a variety of techniques, and so we have no indication whatsoever in the literature which of the extensive list of putative species (e.g., Aβ-derived diffusible ligands, Aβ*56, AβO, annular protofibrils, synthetic oligomers, SDS stable dimers and trimers, etc.) is most relevant [172], while reproducibility between laboratories using the sophisticated and varied techniques has emerged as a near prohibitive problem (Figure 4.2). This issue is not removed by studying oligomers isolated from brain, as isolation creates amyloid fragments. Nevertheless, the linkage of Aβ oligomers with synaptotoxicity (in turn demonstrated by *in vitro* techniques in highly artificial environments) has continued unabated, proving the unsavory truism that the importance and seriousness of the concept trumps the nature of its evidence. In the end, we are left with the following concept: low-n Aβ species, the specifics of which is unclear, produced as a laboratory artifact by a variety of *in vitro* techniques, are toxic to a subcellular junctional complex, itself only amenable to experimental study, as the first manifestation of a neurodegenerative process [11]. Yet the nucleation and ultimate fibrillization of those species bear no discernible neuroanatomical relationship with hallmark lesions, which in turn are poorly specific indicators of disease, i.e., neurotoxicity, and which are seen in large numbers in the cognitively intact elderly. Also noteworthy is the shift in thought from fibrillar amyloid-β as the detergent insoluble, protease resistant and therefore unequivocally neurotoxic species, to low-n amyloid-β species as the detergent soluble, protease-sensitive, and therefore unequivocally neurotoxic species, emphasizing perhaps the identifying characteristic of the postmodern biomedical scientist: his malleability. As "icing on the cake," the fictitious oligomer-synapse paradigm is now viewed by trusting clinicians and even lay public as the substrate for another non-entity concept, mild cognitive impairment (MCI) [11, 173]. Thus, as the concept embedded in the public goes, the oligomer attacks the synapse early in the disease process, resulting in mild cognitive impairment, which progresses to AD.

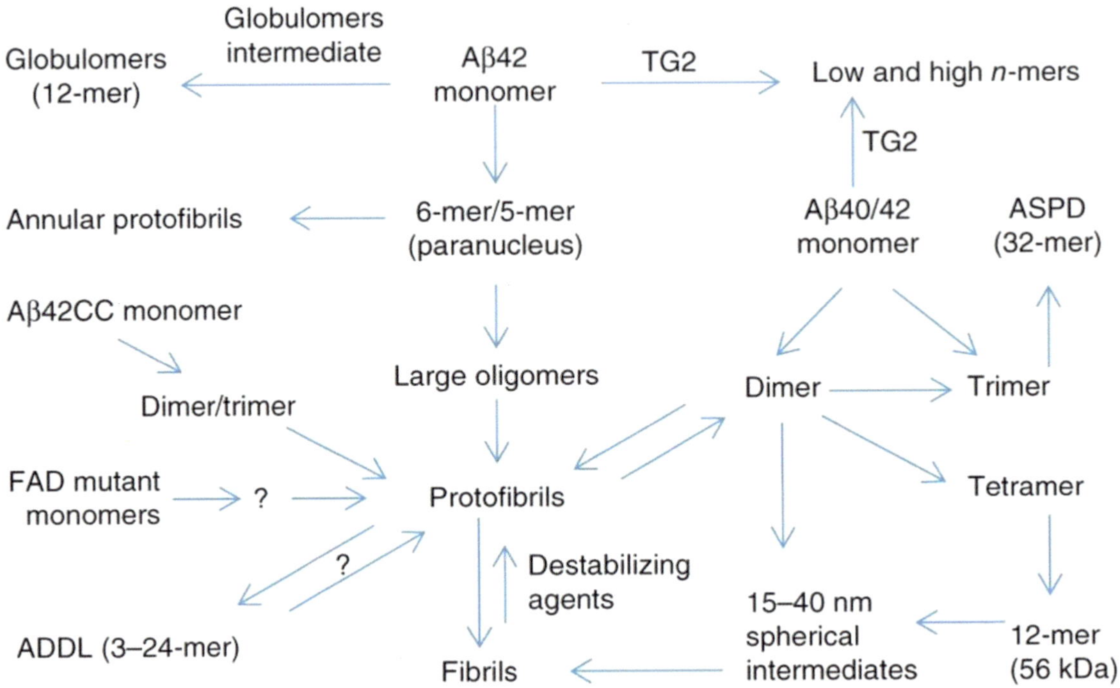

FIGURE 4.2: Schematic diagram demonstrates the complex equilibrium of Aβ monomers, oligomers, and fibrils, and the difficulty inherent in assigning a given protein species to etiology. Used with permission from Benilova et al. [172].

4.3 THE SYNAPSE

Most neuropsychiatric disorders lack a pathological substrate and still affect synaptic function, often profoundly [174]. It is not surprising, therefore, that synaptic alterations are found in aging and in AD. On the other hand, it is commonly stated that "synapse loss is the best correlate of cognitive decline" in AD [175]. What should be kept in mind is that assessment of synaptic damage is entirely investigational and has no diagnostic value in human disease (Figure 4.3). Changes by electron microscopy may be subtle and extremely difficult to quantify. Functional changes in the absence of structural alteration are also likely. Immunohistochemical assessment of synapses via synaptic vesicle proteins synaptophysin or synaptobrevin typically show high background, and are not specific for synapses. As such, synaptic assessment of dementia brains at autopsy, as a means of substantiating a clinical diagnosis, is never done. This is not to say that synaptic integrity should not be a goal in treating neurologic disease, but it is important to be mindful of the presumptions as well as the limitations of studying synapses *in vivo*.

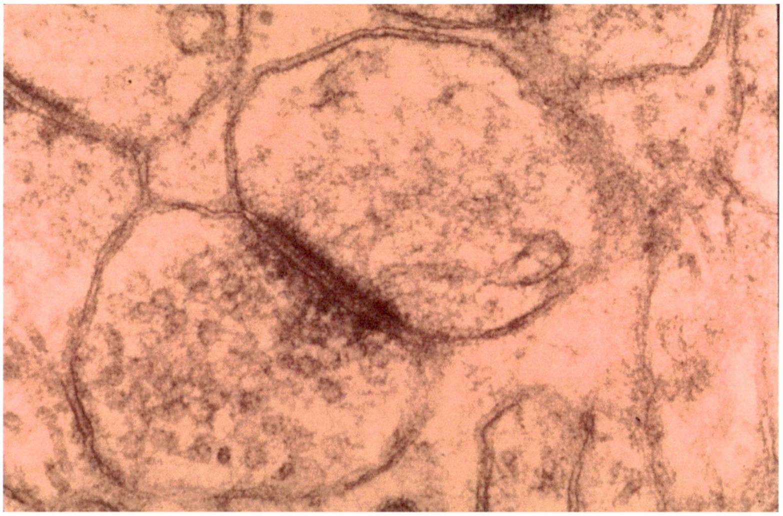

FIGURE 4.3: Transmission electron microscopy of a brain biopsy demonstrates a synapse (junctional complex) with presynaptic and postsynaptic components. While all nervous system disorders involve the synapse, synaptic changes are subtle and nonspecific.

4.4 CLINICOPATHOLOGIC CORRELATIONS

The precept that AD hallmark pathology is a response to disease rather than cause of toxicity predicts that clinicopathological studies approach diminishing returns with mathematical certainty [30]. Response to disease, and variations in response as a function of an infinite number of potential factors, will be rough and imperfect, just like any other chronic disease process in the brain or any other organ system. It is also noteworthy that the task of clinicopathologic correlation in AD, which links clinical disease to pathologic substrate only at end-stage, defies the canonical principle of pathology interpretation, that the more advanced the pathology, the less specific are the changes [13]. In AD, the overwhelming majority of the published experience is interpretation at autopsy, i.e., not merely advanced disease, but by definition end-of-life disease. End-stage pathology, i.e, that pathological expression that indicates the least about etiology, in such cohorts, is the norm.

This overall problem emphasizes the importance of *in vivo* markers of disease, or so-called biomarkers. Although biomarkers are not the focus of the present discussion, Pittsburg Compound B [176], which in essence highlights amyloid (thioflavin binding) by neuro-imaging, has been raised as a potentially important biomarker (Figure 4.4). However, since amyloid correlates weakly with cognition, or not at all in the elderly (see below), the likelihood that this compound could ever be used as a diagnostic test is nil.

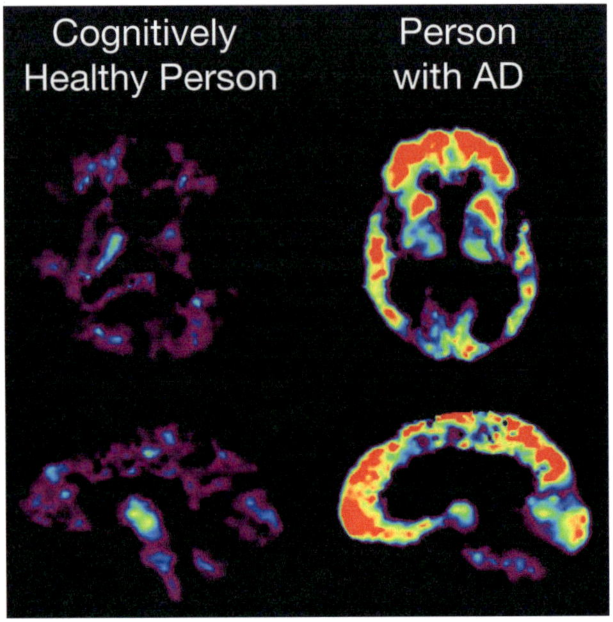

FIGURE 4.4: *In vivo* labeling for thioflavin or amyloid using Pittsburgh Compound B highlights advanced pathology, but is unreliable as a marker of early or preclinical disease.

Nevertheless, numerous clinicopathological studies have been undertaken, under a variety of parameters, endpoints, and study constructs [42, 164, 167, 168, 177–183]. With respect to plaques, correlation between pathology and cognitive status is rough at best, and gets progressively worse as a function of age. Even in the landmark study by Blessed et al. in 1968 [183], a study often touted as the primary piece of clinicopathological data that set the stage for the amyloid cascade, mean plaque counts varied widely for a given cognitive range. This is not particularly surprising given the many subsequent studies and the long known experience with plaque pathology in cognitively normal aged individuals (Figure 4.3), but should objectively argue against Aβ as being etiological.

One of the criticisms of many studies demonstrating limited correlations has been the use of silver impregnation techniques, which is not only technically capricious, but do not accurately distinguish among several plaque types. Neuritic plaques (NP) are considered more disease specific and the more reliable plaque type when attempting to predict dementia, or dysfunction of a cognitive domain subserved by a particular neocortical area, which may in turn be trivialized by less "pathogenic" plaque pathology with indiscriminate staining techniques. Yet the defining feature of the NP, which is the supervening presence of the phospho-tau within dystrophic neurites, is still relegated to second tier status as a pathogenic clue by prevailing wisdom.

The issue of "correlation," which is a low standard when talking about cause, between quantitative plaque pathology and cognition, varies as a function of age. Many studies have now investigated neuropathological changes in the very old, or "oldest old," and come to the same overall conclusion: that plaque pathology is nearly invariable in the very old (Figure 4.5), that elderly can have limited garden variety AD pathology and still be demented, and that application of AD criteria does not reliably distinguish those with dementia from those without [31]. In essence, the clinicopathological paradigm upon which AD pathogenic theories are based, breaks down in senility, suggesting the existence of senile dementia apart from AD.

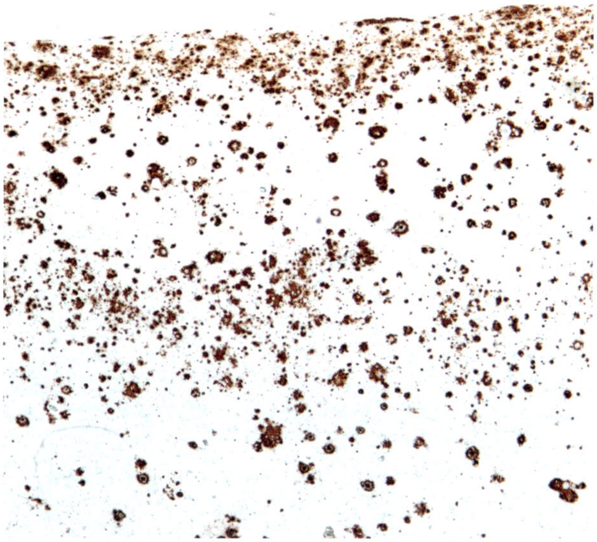

FIGURE 4.5: This low magnification Aβ (4G8) immunostain of frontal cortex was obtained from an autopsy specimen of a 79-year-old man who lived independently with no evidence of cognitive impairment, prior to sudden cardiac death. There is extensive plaque pathology, which is often seen in older subjects without dementia.

The existence of substantial pathology in aged individuals living independently has inspired clinicopathological studies as a function of a number of putative risk and protective factors, one of which is educational attainment. Overall, the data appear to indicate that higher educational attainment, dubiously associated with increased mental activity, is a protective factor [184] (athough this is not uniformly the case [185, 186]), but pathological data may be interpreted in opposite ways. On the one hand, mental activity fosters a healthy brain with lesser degrees of lesion formation and therefore lesser dementia. On the other hand, mental activity may increase "cognitive reserve" such that greater degrees of neuropathology are better tolerated and may stave off cognitive decline. Both are interesting and likely marginal theories with respect to AD. In nun studies, the lack of discernible risk among individuals in a relatively controlled environment, seems to have led to the assessment of more novel risks. In such studies, published in peer reviewed literature, nuns with a lower "idea density" during youth (measured as the number of ideas expressed per 10 words in autobiographies written during youth) [187, 188], fewer teeth [189], and who have failed to be appointed to leadership posts [190], were at increased risk of AD neuropathology.

4.5 PATHOLOGICAL CRITERIA FOR AUTOPSY DIAGNOSIS

4.5.1 KHACHATURIAN CRITERIA

The Khachaturian criteria were the first to emerge, around the same time that Aβ and phospho-tau were being purified from human brain [191]. The criteria recognized the existence of pathology simply with age, and likewise required more advanced pathology with increasing age in order to qualify for AD. Specifically, plaques were counted on the basis of number per 200x microscopic field, with two to five plaques per field for patients age 50 and younger, eight or more per field for patients age 50–65, greater than ten per field for patients age 66-75, and greater than fifteen per field for patients older than 75. Tangles were generally considered less critical and specifically not required for diagnosis, perhaps because of the emerging evidence surrounding the genetics of Aβ and Down syndrome. Interestingly, the degree with which clinical history impacted the diagnosis was a matter of some debate, although it was agreed that:

> *"In the presence of a positive clinical history of AD these criteria should be revised downwards, although to what extent remains to be determined by further research. One suggestion was that one might only need 50% as many lesions in neocortical samples to retain a high confidence for the histological diagnosis"* [191].

These two sentences appropriately summarize the problem of clinicopathological correlation that continues to the present.

4.5.2 BRAAK STAGING

In 1991, Braak and Braak studied neurodegenerative pathology at autopsy in 83 subjects [164]. The Braak study was an intermingling of aging and dementia, as fewer than half of the subjects were clinically demented during life. Both plaque pathology and neurofibrillary pathology were staged, although there was frank admission of considerable inter-individual variation in amyloid accumulation in lesser-affected brains, and a constant pattern of amyloid accumulation in end-stage (the latter was not invariably associated with clinical dementia). More noteworthy in the Braak study was a predictable, stepwise progression of neurofibrillary pathology from a so-called transentorhinal stages (I and II), to a limbic stages (III and IV), to isocortical stage (V and VI) (Figure 4.6). None of the transentorhinal stage subjects were demented during life, whereas all of the isocortical stage subjects were demented, along with about half of the limbic stage subjects. Although cognitive details were sparse, neuroanatomical characterization was rigorous, and convincingly demonstrated the eloquence with which phospho-tau accumulates as a function of time and cognition, and equally the nonspecificity with which Aβ accumulates as a function of the same.

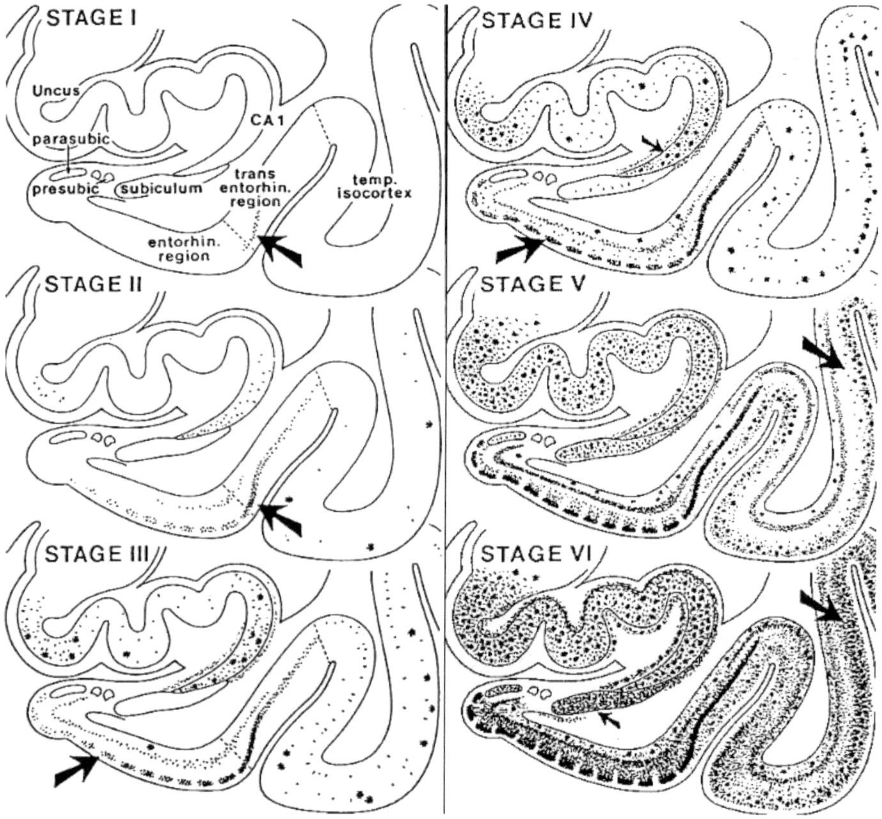

FIGURE 4.6: Schematic diagram of Braak stages of neurofibrillary pathology, modified from Braak and Braak, 1991 [178]. Braak staging was undertaken in subjects with and without evidence of dementia during life, representing an intermingling of age and disease. Nevertheless, it shows a stepwise progression of neurofibrillary degeneration as a function of age and dementia. Examination for plaque pathology was performed in the same study; however, plaque pathology was variable early in disease, and nonspecific late.

4.5.3 CERAD (CONSORTIUM TO ESTABLISH A REGISTRY FOR ALZHEIMER'S DISEASE) GUIDELINES

Around the same time, a consortium of clinicians from 15 Alzheimer's Disease centers met to develop, among other things, consensus neuropathological criteria for AD [42]. CERAD chose the neuritic plaque as the defining neuropathological feature, and used a semiquantitative approach (sparse versus moderate versus frequent) of a limited number of brain regions, to facilitate interobserver agreement, overall ease of interpretation, and databasing (Figure 4.7). It is interesting that CERAD recommended the silver impregnation technique, despite well-known technical difficulties as well as lack of efficacy in distinguishing the neuritic plaque from other plaque subtypes (particularly since the neuropathology component was based entirely on the neuritic plaque). CERAD further added a clinical history component to the algorithm, and like the precursor Khachaturian approach, further qualified the pathological assessment into subcategories as a function of age. Thus, the combined clinical and pathological data were assigned possible, probably, and definite AD.

CERAD Guidelines

Plaque Frequency

Age	None	Sparse	Moderate	Frequent
<50	0	C	C	C
50-75	0	B	C	C
>75	0	A	B	C

0 = no evidence of AD; A = uncertain; B = suggestive of AD; C = indicative of AD

"Definite AD" = C plus clinical dementia
"Probably AD" = B plus clinical dementia
"Possible AD" = A plus clinical dementia, or B or C and no dementia

FIGURE 4.7: CERAD (Consortium to Establish a Registry for Alzheimer's Disease) criteria for AD from 1991 emphasized neuritic plaques as well as age, and the presence or absence of dementia [42]. The concept that older individuals require more extensive pathology for diagnostic specificity is prima facie evidence of lack of toxicity of pathological lesions.

4.5.4 NIA-REAGAN CRITERIA

NIA-Reagan guidelines simply presumed congruity between advanced stages of Braak and advanced assessment by CERAD, and combined the two, to yield "high likelihood," "intermediate likelihood," and "low likelihood" categories [192]. The descriptive terminology used in the

NIA-Reagan guidelines is particularly illustrative of the bias that is pervasive in AD research, by stating that the various likelihoods that dementia are "due to Alzheimer's Disease lesions," i.e., lesions are toxic. This is evidently offered, interestingly enough, while invoking CERAD guidelines that forgive an extent of pathology in older individuals, implying rather directly that the older brain tolerates neurotoxic lesions better than the younger brain. If nothing else, the early attempts at consensus criteria are an indicator of the difficulties with which disease is assessed as a function of hallmark lesions. This further suggests to us that neuropathology of AD is a reactive phenomenon, and that only the broadest correlations are possible, as would be expected in chronic, non-neoplastic neurodegeneration that overlaps substantially with the aging process.

4.5.5 2012 CRITERIA

Fifteen years after NIA-Reagan combined CERAD and Braak, clinicians from various centers met again to further refine the diagnostic criteria for AD, espousing a "practical approach" to a complex issue [193] and the most complicated set of recommendations to date (Figure 4.8). The updated set of criteria are ironically given the acronym ABC criteria, referring to the amyloid staging by Thal et al. [194], Braak staging [164], and CERAD assessment of NP frequency [42]. Thal and Braak stages are simplified from 5 and 6 stages respectively, to three each, and the tripartite assessment is fed into a table, yielding an extent of "AD neuropathologic change." As a practical matter, a close analysis of the table indicates that strong correlations with dementia are only possible with the most advanced pathology. Moreover, the long known problems surrounding the inclusion of clinical signs into the autopsy diagnosis are discarded wholesale, as history of dementia plays no role in the assessment. "AD neuropathologic change," accompanied by different degrees of pathology for A, B, and C, becomes the final interpretation.

2012 Criteria of Alzheimer Disease (ABC METHOD)

"A"	Thal Phase for plaques [57]	"B"	Braak and Braak NFT Stage [14, 15]	"C"	CERAD neuritic plaque score [41]
0		0	None	0	None
1	1 or 2	1	I or II	1	Sparse
2	3	2	III or IV	2	Moderate
3	4 or 5	3	V or VI	3	Frequent

AD Neuropathologic Change		B		
A[2]	C[3]	0 or 1	2	3
0	0	Not[4]	Not[4]	Not[4]
1	0 or 1	Low	Low	Low[5]
1	2 or 3[7]	Low	Intermediate	Intermediate[5]
2	Any C	Low[6]	Intermediate	Intermediate[5]
3	0 or 1	Low[6]	Intermediate	Intermediate[5]
3	2 or 3	Low[6]	Intermediate	High

FIGURE 4.8: 2012 guidelines for Alzheimer's Disease neuropathologic change combined amyloid staging by Thal [194], Braak neurofibrillary stage [164], and CERAD neuritic plaque scores [193]. The data are fed into a table and an overall extent of change is determined. The lower table further indicates the likelihood that dementia could be associated with Alzheimer's Disease neuropathological change, on the basis of the criteria. Noteworthy is that while a likelihood of dementia may be inferred from the table, clinical data were not a component of the criteria. It is also interesting that the likelihood of agreement between AD change and dementia was "high" only if Braak stage and the amyloid scores were most advanced.

The issues surrounding assignment of diagnosis to a given brain are not trivial for the molecular biologist. The rigorous study of brain tissue at the molecular level requires rigorous characterization of the pathology, and a level of certainty that the tissue in question is an accurate representation of the disease under study. What should be kept in mind from all of these studies is that AD is in many respects a diagnosis of exclusion [13]. The changes associated with AD overlap extensively with age, and the overlap is more so than any other age related neurodegenerative process. Indeed, neurodegenerative conditions apart from AD (e.g., Lewy body dementia, frontotemporal dementia, various tauopathies, Huntington disease, amyotrophic lateral sclerosis) are reasonably specific for the clinical condition in the absence of any clinical data, and are much less likely to be confused with simple aging. AD on the other hand requires an extreme quantitative level of otherwise age-related lesions for diagnostic certainty. To this point, Nelson et al., carried out an interesting study of Braak stage VI AD cases [195]. In this study, the authors found that the level of cognition tended to correlate with NFT count, even within this advanced stage subgroup. What this indicates is that neuropathological diagnosis of AD at autopsy is most certain, and one could even argue that it is *only* certain, when the pathology is end-stage (Figure 4.9). Short of Braak VI, other co-morbidities should be sought (vascular disease, Lewy bodies, polypharmacy, etc.) before concluding that tissue in question is from a genuine AD brain. To be sure, the most illustrative AD pathology, and that extent of pathology that is most predictable of dementia during life, is also the most downstream. Such might be among the considerations for the molecular neuroscientist when attempting to translate cellular or preclinical data to human tissue.

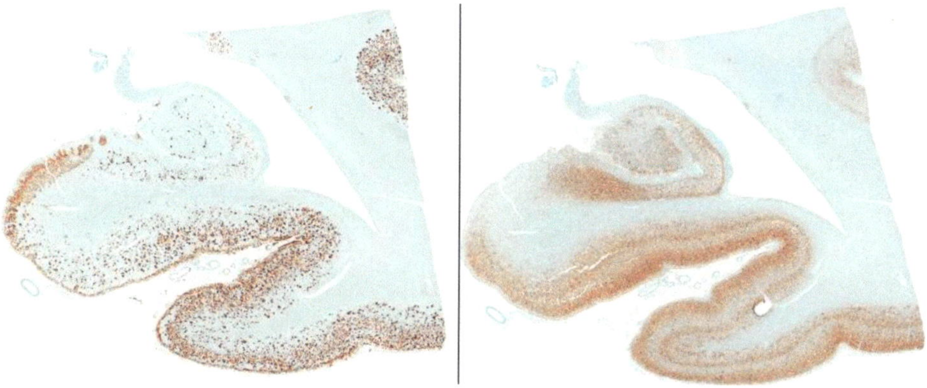

FIGURE 4.9: Low magnification photomicrographs of hippocampus and adjacent medial temporal lobe structures immunostained for Aβ (4G8), left, and phospho-tau (AT8), right, show an abundance of plaques and neurofibrillary degeneration. The changes represent Braak stage VI [164], "definite" AD by CERAD criteria [42], and AD neuropathologic change A3/B3/C3 by 2012 criteria [204]. The changes are convincing for the presence of antemortem cognitive function indicative of AD. Any lesser degree of pathology, however, is accompanied by greater uncertainty in the diagnosis and should raise the possibility of co-morbid conditions affecting cognition, such as vascular disease and Lewy body dementia.

CHAPTER 5

Synopsis and Conclusions

Detailed study of the molecular pathology of Alzheimer's Disease reinforces humility before nature. Molecular pathogenesis began with a circumspect appraisal of the correlation between clinical disease and morphologic changes, and it continues over a century later with a circumspect appraisal of the correlation between clinical disease and molecular pathways. Optimism for the future, while still apparent, is guarded. It is guarded not because of a limited extent of new knowledge of molecular changes in AD. Indeed, new knowledge is extensive, and in many instances has opened up new areas of investigation and novel biological phenomena not previously described in humans. Rather, optimism is guarded because this exponential expansion of data is accompanied by an utter inability to alter the cognitive trajectory in AD. The inability, moreover, postdates many dozens of clinical trials, each with expressed enthusiasm for therapeutic intervention.

The enthusiasm, for its part, has been remarkable. The number of scholarly papers in the AD field espousing "therapeutic implications" number in the thousands. Grant applications in the AD field not only profess the same, but even demonstrate therapeutic benefit in preclinical studies again and again. Strict attention is paid among funding agencies to translational neurobiology, as each agency rather impatiently requires promise for "bench to bedside" results. Peer reviewers and study sections routinely tout the importance of amyloid while criticizing studies for lack of a hypothesis and for going against the prevailing arguments made based on molecular data. The world's most prestigious scientific publications eagerly print the most prescient and therapy-centered primary data, and then solicit scholarly reviews on the latest breakthrough from esteemed laboratories—laboratories that populate the most elite academic institutions, with decorated histories of publications, citations, financial support, partnership with private industry, patents, and appearances in popular media. Therapeutic intervention is within our grasp, it would seem, if only we would reach out to seize it.

Yet despite countless breakthroughs in the elucidation of the amyloid cascade, the cognitive trajectory in AD is no different today than the day AD was described in 1906. Medical science has not laid a glove on the disorder that afflicts millions of Americans and is anticipated to afflict millions more at an even higher percentage in the future. The only remotely beneficial, and entirely palliative, therapeutic option rests, interestingly enough, in the enhancement of cholinergic transmission or lifestyle intervention, having nothing to do with pathogenic proteins and putative, linear cascades.

How can this be? The answer may lie in the fundamental misinterpretation of chronic disease. A simple thought experiment with a 100-year-old mindset may be a case in point. Alzheimer's Described AD lesions in an autopsy specimen, from a patient who had experienced cognitive deterioration for a number of years. Among the competing diagnoses of that era were general paresis, which was indeed a chronic condition but with ultimately a clear-cut infectious etiology. The parenchymal pathology of general paresis consists of microglial activation, which, if perceived as etiological, might have been targeted for therapy and have predictably failed, since etiology, or infection by *Treponema pallidum*, would have gone unaddressed. The other major diagnostic consideration for the cognitive decline of Auguste D. was cerebrovascular arterial sclerosis, a condition with which Alzheimer was intimately familiar. Likewise, had this been the underlying disease, and had the proliferating fibroblasts in the walls of cerebral blood vessels been targeted, the systemic etiological factors, including hypertensive vascular disease, diabetes mellitus, and/or hyperlipidemia, or potential cardiac etiologies for ischemic complications, would have gone unaddressed, and end organ complications would have no doubt continued.

The analogies go on in systemic diseases. If one attempts to treat interstitial lung disease by targeting interstitial collagen, or chronic kidney disease by targeting sclerotic glomeruli, or chronic liver disease by targeting bridging fibrosis, or chronic neuromuscular disease by targeting fibrofatty ingrowth, etiology goes on unaddressed, and success depends on the likelihood that ameliorating a disease response, which from an evolutionary perspective may be a beneficial response, will assuage the deleterious molecular events leading to disease.

AD is no different from the standpoint of a chronic, non-neoplastic disease process. It differs in that, for reasons peculiar to the brain and the difficulties of studying the pathology of neurodegeneration during life, AD is defined by the end-stage pathology. Likewise, innumerable clinicopathologic studies indicate that the appearance of Aβ of whatever species, be it monomer, low-n mer, protofibril, or fibrillar amyloid in diffuse, cored, or neuritic plaques, is a late event and is more likely a response to a systems pathobiology, the knowledge of which is in its infancy. Phospho-tau accumulation, although much more eloquent than Aβ in its relationship with clinical disease, is a manifestly reactive phenomenon. So the conclusion is clear, both in theory and in reality from clinical trials: targeting adaptive pathological proteins and chronic disease not only does not work, but may be harmful.

The molecular pathologist may also keep in mind that elaboration of Aβ within the human brain is a physiological process. Much has been made about the relative significance of the Aβ42 species as a pathogenic mediator, and increased in the Aβ42/Aβ40 ratio in, for example, familial AD. Even in this instance, however, an absolute increase in Aβ42 has been challenged as mentioned about, and a close look at some kindreds even indicates an overall reduction in Aβ. The same is true of Down syndrome. Toxicity of Aβ42, while embedded in the literature, not to mention the minds of scientists and lay people alike, has yet to be demonstrated *in vivo*.

Moreover, Aβ involvement in disease has clearly been oversimplified. The basic process of γ-secretase cleavage, for example, involves a catalytic site, diverse subunits, and regulatory factors about which almost nothing is known. AβPP itself has multiple domains and a promoter sequence indicating a generalized housekeeping receptor, whose function is elusive but nevertheless extends beyond Aβ synthesis. AβPP bears striking orthology to proteins such as Notch, involved in development of lower organisms, utilizing strikingly similar enzyme cleavages for cellular signaling and recycling, including essentially the same evolutionarily conserved catalytic site of γ-secretase. Aβ itself may play an important role in signal transduction and transcriptional activation during life. Other beneficial roles such as binding of transition metals and blunting oxidative stress in the brain have already been demonstrated [196]. Yet somehow in aging and in disease, Aβ synthesis is said to be a "rate limiting" effector of synaptotoxicity, singularly changing its metabolic activity in favor of neurodegeneration, and against the host organism and millions of years of evolution.

Nevertheless, lesion targeting continues unabated. There are many reasons for this, the most benign of which is the power of central dogma as a governing concept in biology. The notion of "Familial AD," having AβPP mutations (gene-protein-disease) or presenilin mutations (enzyme-substrate-disease), has the appeal of elegance and simplicity, adhering to central dogma while providing a singular (some would say reductionist) molecular explanation for disease. When viewed in the abstract, or with only casual understanding of the neuropathology, the perseveration on the amyloid cascade is as attractive and it is understandable.

A more careful appraisal, however, identifies germline, pathogenic mutation as an aberration, one that sets up a fundamentally different, diseased, and anti-Darwinian cellular milieu. Even then, it should be noted that the deleterious environment exists for decades with no discernible clinical or pathological changes, prior to the onset of neurodegeneration. It seems that the human proteome, comprised of thousands of actively translated proteins within neurons [197], trivializes the effects of a pathogenic mutation for many years, even decades. Therefore, using familial disease as an equivalent of sporadic disease, and in turn assigning the pathogenesis of disease to the effects of a single protein of normal primary structure, fails to take into account the whole of the cell, to say nothing of the whole organism. Here again, we should be reminded that transgenic models used in preclinical studies are based on pathogenic mutation, i.e., familial disease, and yet clinical trials, justified on the basis of the data obtained from transgenic constructs, are applied to the sporadic milieu. Trial failures were thus predictable and should not be surprising [198].

AD research is also hampered by external factors that bring into the conversation the unsavory and yet ubiquitous issues of money and politics. AD affects millions of individuals, and at an enormous cost to society. It is estimated that by 2050, AD will affect over 13 million Americans at a cost of over 1 trillion dollars per year (http://www.alz.org/). The market for a therapeutic, and the associated profits, is in place and waiting watchfully. Private industry is working feverishly for a product, as it means billions of dollars virtually overnight. It is no secret that the bulk of the resources are dedicated toward a therapeutic that follows the amyloid cascade hypothesis in lockstep. To the credit of the American system favoring evidence-based medicine, clinical trials have to date not been significantly manipulated, and efficacy has not been demonstrated where it did not exist. The amount of money at stake and the extent of the conflict of interests have not been without casualties.

Probably more pervasive, however is genuine bias. The system of public funding of research requires the researcher to embrace narrow molecular constructs, and promote those constructs successfully to granting agencies. Such is a blueprint for *a priori* bias, politicking, and the unconscious data analysis bias when one's career and family security depend on its ultimate success.

A broader philosophical question is how one assesses the start of the art. The history of science is marked by such flawed concepts as humoral theory, blood letting, craniometry, and eugenics just to name a few. All were promoted and practiced by the world's elite physicians and scientists of their eras, and were endorsed by the world's finest academic institutions. So the question is this: do we view the current state of knowledge from the modern perspective, and pat ourselves on the back for the extensive knowledge of molecular biology we now enjoy, or do we see ourselves from the standpoint of 100 years hence, when today's science will, with absolute certainty, be regarded as naïve and utterly primitive?

As we look back, we may admire Alzheimer and his contemporaries for seminal histopathological observations, but Alzheimer himself should be more admired for his humility and objectivity about this own data, rare gifts afforded to him by his God-given personality traits. Perhaps the luxury of a supportive spouse as well, allowed him to follow a course directed by the data and nothing else, and kept him from pursuing full-time clinical medicine, or perhaps using his skills to devise and sell treatment approaches with no real hope for therapeutic benefit (see clinicaltrials.gov).

References

1. Alzheimer A. Über eine eigenartige Erkrankung der Hirnrinde. *Allg Zeitschr Psychiatr* 1907;64:146-8.
2. Berchtold NC, Cotman CW. Evolution in the conceptualization of dementia and Alzheimer's Disease: Greco-Roman period to the 1960s. *Neurobiol Aging* 1998;19:173-89. DOI: 10.1016/S0197-4580(98)00052-9.
3. Konrad Maurer UM. *The life of a physician and the career of a disease*. New York: Columbia University Press; 2003. DOI: 10.1002/gps.1036.
4. Alzheimer A. Über eigenartige Krankheitsfälle des späteren Alters. *Zeitschr Gesamte Neurol Psychiatr* 1911;4:356-85. DOI: 10.1007/BF02866241.
5. Kraepelin E. Kraepelin E. Psychiatrie. *Klinische Psychiatrie.* Leipzig: Barth; ; 1910.
6. Moller HJ, Graeber MB. The case described by Alois Alzheimer in 1911. Historical and conceptual perspectives based on the clinical record and neurohistological sections. *Eur Arch Psychiatry Clin Neurosci* 1998;248:111-22.
7. Bielschowsky M. Die Silberimprägnation der Achsencylinder. *Neurologisches Zentralblatt*, Leipzig 1902;21:579-84.
8. Herrup K. Reimagining Alzheimer's Disease--an age-based hypothesis. *J Neurosci* 2010;30:16755-62. DOI: 10.1523/JNEUROSCI.4521-10.2010.
9. Selkoe DJ. Alzheimer's Disease. *Cold Spring Harb Perspect Biol* 2012;3.
10. Castellani RJ, Perry G. Pathogenesis and disease-modifying therapy in Alzheimer's Disease: the flat line of progress. *Arch Med Res* 2012;43:694-8. DOI: 10.1016/j.arcmed.2012.09.009.
11. Castellani RJ, Smith MA. Compounding artefacts with uncertainty, and an amyloid cascade hypothesis that is 'too big to fail'. *J Pathol* 2011;224:147-52. DOI: 10.1002/path.2885.
12. Bielschowsky M. *Cytology and Cellular Pathology of the Nervous System*. Montreal, Canada: Paul B. Hoeber, Inc; 1932.
13. Castellani RJ, Lee HG, Zhu X, Perry G, Smith MA. Alzheimer's Disease pathology as a host response. *J Neuropathol Exp Neurol* 2008;67:523-31. DOI: 10.1097/NEN.0b013e318177eaf4.

14. Blocq P, Marinesco, G. Sur les le´ sions et la pathoge´ nie de l'e´ pilepsie dite essentielle. *Sem Med* 1892;12:445-6.
15. Beljahow S. Pathological modifications in the brains of demented patients. *J Ment Sci* 18889;35:261-2.
16. Redlich E. Uber miliare Sklerose der Hirnrinde bei seniler Atrophie. *Psychiat Neurol* 1989;17:208-16.
17. Miyake K. Beitra¨ ge zur Kenntnis der Altersvera¨ nderungen der menschlichen Hirnrinde. *Obersteiner's Arb* 1906;13:212-59.
18. Goedert M. Oskar Fischer and the study of dementia. *Brain* 2009;132:1102-11. DOI: 10.1093/brain/awn256.
19. Fischer O. Miliare Nekrosen mit drusigen Wucherungen der Neurofibrillen, eine regelma¨ ssige Vera¨ nderung der Hirnrinde bei seniler Demenz. Monatsschr *Psychiat Neurol* 1907;22:361-72. DOI: 10.1159/000211873.
20. Fischer O. Die presbyophrene Demenz, deren anatomische Grundlage und klinische Abgrenzung. *Z ges Neurol Psychiat* 1910;3:371-471. DOI: 10.1007/BF02893605.
21. Fuller SC. A study of miliary plaques found in the brains of the aged. *Am J Insanity* 1911;68:147-234.
22. Bonfiglio F. Di speciali reperti in uno caso di probabile sifilide cerebrale. *Rev Sper Freniatr* 1908;34:196-206.
23. Perusini G. U¨ ber klinisch und histologisch eigenartige psychische Erkrankungen des spa¨ teren Lebensalters. *Nissl-Alzheimers Histol Histopathol Arb Hirnr* 1909;3:297-351.
24. Sarteschi U. Contributo all'istologia patologica della presbiofrenia. *Riv Sper Freniatr* 1909;35:464-84.
25. Yu CE, Marchani E, Nikisch G, et al. The N141I mutation in PSEN2: implications for the quintessential case of Alzheimer's Disease. *Arch Neurol* 2010;67:631-3. DOI: 10.1001/archneurol.2010.87.
26. Muller U, Winter P, Graeber MB. Alois Alzheimer's case, Auguste D., did not carry the N141I mutation in PSEN2 characteristic of Alzheimer's Disease in Volga Germans. *Arch Neurol* 2011;68:1210-1, author reply 1. DOI: 10.1001/archneurol.2011.218.
27. Muller U, Winter P, Graeber MB. A presenilin 1 mutation in the first case of Alzheimer's Disease. *Lancet Neurol* 2013;12:129-30. DOI: 10.1016/S1474-4422(12)70307-1.
28. Klunemann HH, Fronhofer W, Werner-Fuchtenbusch D, et al. Characterization of the kindred of Alois Alzheimer's patient with plaque-only dementia. *Alzheimer Dis Assoc Disord* 2006;20:291-4. DOI: 10.1097/01.wad.0000213855.81989.c8.

29. Holmes C, Boche D, Wilkinson D, et al. Long-term effects of Abeta42 immunisation in Alzheimer's Disease: follow-up of a randomised, placebo-controlled phase I trial. *Lancet* 2008;372:216-23. DOI: 10.1016/S0140-6736(08)61075-2.
30. Nelson PT, Alafuzoff I, Bigio EH, et al. Correlation of Alzheimer's Disease neuropathologic changes with cognitive status: a review of the literature. *J Neuropathol Exp Neurol* 2011;71:362-81. DOI: 10.1097/NEN.0b013e31825018f7.
31. Driscoll I, Resnick SM, Troncoso JC, An Y, O'Brien R, Zonderman AB. Impact of Alzheimer's pathology on cognitive trajectories in nondemented elderly. *Ann Neurol* 2006;60:688-95. DOI: 10.1002/ana.21031.
32. Hardy JA, Higgins GA. Alzheimer's Disease: the amyloid cascade hypothesis. *Science* 1992;256:184-5. DOI: 10.1126/science.1566067.
33. Castellani R.J., Alexiev, B.A., Phillips, D., Perry, G., Smith, M.A. Microscopic Investigations in Neurodegenerative Diseases. In: A Mendez Vilas JD, ed. *Modern Research and Investigation Topics in Microscopy: Formatex*; 2007:172-82.
34. Yamamoto T., Hirano A. A comparative study of modified Bielschowsky, Bodian and thioflavin S stains on Alzheimer's neurofibrillary tangles. *Neuropathol Appl Neurobiol* 1986;12:3-9. DOI: 10.1111/j.1365-2990.1986.tb00677.x.
35. Divry P. Etude histo-chimique des plaques seniles. *J Belge Neurol Psychiatr*;. 27 1927:643-57.
36. Armstrong RA. Beta-amyloid plaques: stages in life history or independent origin? *Dement Geriatr Cogn Disord* 1998;9:227-38. DOI: 10.1159/000017051.
37. James Lowe SSM, Bradley T Hyman, Dennis W Dickson. Aging and Dementia. In: Jellinger KA, ed. Greenfield's *Neuropathology*. London: Edward Arnold Ltd; 2008:1048-58.
38. Brooks WS, Kwok JB, Kril JJ, et al. Alzheimer's Disease with spastic paraparesis and 'cotton wool' plaques: two pedigrees with PS-1 exon 9 deletions. *Brain* 2003;126:783-91. DOI: 10.1093/brain/awg084.
39. Le TV, Crook R, Hardy J, Dickson DW. Cotton wool plaques in non-familial late-onset Alzheimer's Disease. *J Neuropathol Exp Neurol* 2001;60:1051-61.
40. Suenaga T, Hirano A, Llena JF, Ksiezak-Reding H, Yen SH, Dickson DW. Modified Bielschowsky and immunocytochemical studies on cerebellar plaques in Alzheimer's Disease. *J Neuropathol Exp Neurol* 1990;49:31-40. DOI: 10.1097/00005072-199001000-00004.
41. Rifenburg RP, Perry G. Dystrophic neurites define diffuse as well as core-containing senile plaques in Alzheimer's Disease. *Neurodegeneration* 1995;4:235-7.

42. Mirra SS, Heyman A, McKeel D, et al. The Consortium to Establish a Registry for Alzheimer's Disease (CERAD). Part II. Standardization of the neuropathologic assessment of Alzheimer's Disease. *Neurology* 1991;41:479-86. DOI: 10.1212/WNL.41.4.479.
43. Glenner GG, Wong CW. Alzheimer's Disease and Down's syndrome: sharing of a unique cerebrovascular amyloid fibril protein. *Biochem Biophys Res Commun* 1984;122:1131-5. DOI: 10.1016/0006-291X(84)91209-9.
44. Kang J, Lemaire HG, Unterbeck A, et al. The precursor of Alzheimer's Disease amyloid A4 protein resembles a cell-surface receptor. *Nature* 1987;325:733-6. DOI: 10.1038/325733a0.
45. Robakis NK, Ramakrishna N, Wolfe G, Wisniewski HM. Molecular cloning and characterization of a cDNA encoding the cerebrovascular and the neuritic plaque amyloid peptides. *Proc Natl Acad Sci U S A* 1987;84:4190-4. DOI: 10.1073/pnas.84.12.4190.
46. Goldgaber D, Lerman MI, McBride OW, Saffiotti U, Gajdusek DC. Characterization and chromosomal localization of a cDNA encoding brain amyloid of Alzheimer's Disease. *Science* 1987;235:877-80. DOI: 10.1126/science.3810169.
47. Tanzi RE, Gusella JF, Watkins PC, et al. Amyloid beta protein gene: cDNA, mRNA distribution, and genetic linkage near the Alzheimer locus. *Science* 1987;235:880-4. DOI: 10.1126/science.2949367.
48. Lemaire HG, Salbaum JM, Multhaup G, et al. The PreA4(695) precursor protein of Alzheimer's Disease A4 amyloid is encoded by 16 exons. *Nucleic Acids Res* 1989;17:517-22. DOI: 10.1093/nar/17.2.517.
49. Yoshikai S, Sasaki H, Doh-ura K, Furuya H, Sakaki Y. Genomic organization of the human amyloid beta-protein precursor gene. *Gene* 1990;87:257-63. DOI: 10.1016/0378-1119(90)90310-N.
50. Tanzi RE, McClatchey AI, Lamperti ED, Villa-Komaroff L, Gusella JF, Neve RL. Protease inhibitor domain encoded by an amyloid protein precursor mRNA associated with Alzheimer's Disease. *Nature* 1988;331:528-30. DOI: 10.1038/331528a0.
51. Kitaguchi N, Takahashi Y, Tokushima Y, Shiojiri S, Ito H. Novel precursor of Alzheimer's Disease amyloid protein shows protease inhibitory activity. *Nature* 1988;331:530-2. DOI: 10.1038/331530a0.
52. Ponte P, Gonzalez-DeWhitt P, Schilling J, et al. A new A4 amyloid mRNA contains a domain homologous to serine proteinase inhibitors. *Nature* 1988;331:525-7. DOI: 10.1038/331525a0.
53. Clark MJ, Gagnon J, Williams AF, Barclay AN. MRC OX-2 antigen: a lymphoid/neuronal membrane glycoprotein with a structure like a single immunoglobulin light chain. *EMBO J* 1985;4:113-8.

54. Haass C, Kaether C, Thinakaran G, Sisodia S. Trafficking and proteolytic processing of APP. *Cold Spring Harb Perspect Med* 2012;2:a006270. DOI: 10.1101/cshperspect.a006270.
55. Venugopal C, Demos CM, Rao KS, Pappolla MA, Sambamurti K. Beta-secretase: structure, function, and evolution. *CNS Neurol Disord Drug Targets* 2008;7:278-94. DOI: 10.2174/187152708784936626.
56. Lin X, Koelsch G, Wu S, Downs D, Dashti A, Tang J. Human aspartic protease memapsin 2 cleaves the beta-secretase site of beta-amyloid precursor protein. *Proc Natl Acad Sci U S A* 2000;97:1456-60. DOI: 10.1073/pnas.97.4.1456.
57. Hussain I, Powell DJ, Howlett DR, et al. ASP1 (BACE2) cleaves the amyloid precursor protein at the beta-secretase site. *Mol Cell Neurosci* 2000;16:609-19. DOI: 10.1006/mcne.2000.0884.
58. Yan R, Bienkowski MJ, Shuck ME, et al. Membrane-anchored aspartyl protease with Alzheimer's Disease beta-secretase activity. *Nature* 1999;402:533-7. DOI: 10.1038/990107.
59. Vassar R, Bennett BD, Babu-Khan S, et al. Beta-secretase cleavage of Alzheimer's amyloid precursor protein by the transmembrane aspartic protease BACE. *Science* 1999;286:735-41. DOI: 10.1126/science.286.5440.735.
60. Sinha S, Anderson JP, Barbour R, et al. Purification and cloning of amyloid precursor protein beta-secretase from human brain. *Nature* 1999;402:537-40. DOI: 10.1038/990114.
61. Sinha S, Knops J, Esch F, Moyer ED, Oltersdorf T. Conversion of the Alzheimer's beta-amyloid precursor protein (APP) Kunitz domain into a potent human neutrophil elastase inhibitor. *J Biol Chem* 1991;266:21011-3.
62. Solans A, Estivill X, de La Luna S. A new aspartyl protease on 21q22.3, BACE2, is highly similar to Alzheimer's amyloid precursor protein beta-secretase. *Cytogenet Cell Genet* 2000;89:177-84. DOI: 10.1159/000015608.
63. Cai XD, Golde TE, Younkin SG. Release of excess amyloid beta protein from a mutant amyloid beta protein precursor. *Science* 1993;259:514-6. DOI: 10.1126/science.8424174.
64. Gruninger-Leitch F, Schlatter D, Kung E, Nelbock P, Dobeli H. Substrate and inhibitor profile of BACE (beta-secretase) and comparison with other mammalian aspartic proteases. *J Biol Chem* 2002;277:4687-93. DOI: 10.1074/jbc.M109266200.
65. Tomasselli AG, Qahwash I, Emmons TL, et al. Employing a superior BACE1 cleavage sequence to probe cellular APP processing. *J Neurochem* 2003;84:1006-17. DOI: 10.1046/j.1471-4159.2003.01597.x.
66. He X, Li F, Chang WP, Tang J. GGA proteins mediate the recycling pathway of memapsin 2 (BACE). *J Biol Chem* 2005;280:11696-703. DOI: 10.1074/jbc.M411296200.

67. He X, Zhu G, Koelsch G, Rodgers KK, Zhang XC, Tang J. Biochemical and structural characterization of the interaction of memapsin 2 (beta-secretase) cytosolic domain with the VHS domain of GGA proteins. *Biochemistry* 2003;42:12174-80. DOI: 10.1021/bi035199h.
68. Walter J, Fluhrer R, Hartung B, et al. Phosphorylation regulates intracellular trafficking of beta-secretase. *J Biol Chem* 2001;276:14634-41. DOI: 10.1074/jbc.M011116200.
69. Benjannet S, Elagoz A, Wickham L, et al. Post-translational processing of beta-secretase (beta-amyloid-converting enzyme) and its ectodomain shedding. The pro- and transmembrane/cytosolic domains affect its cellular activity and amyloid-beta production. *J Biol Chem* 2001;276:10879-87. DOI: 10.1074/jbc.M009899200.
70. Haniu M, Denis P, Young Y, et al. Characterization of Alzheimer's beta -secretase protein BACE. A pepsin family member with unusual properties. *J Biol Chem* 2000;275:21099-106. DOI: 10.1074/jbc.M002095200.
71. Huse JT, Pijak DS, Leslie GJ, Lee VM, Doms RW. Maturation and endosomal targeting of beta-site amyloid precursor protein-cleaving enzyme. The Alzheimer's Disease beta-secretase. *J Biol Chem* 2000;275:33729-37. DOI: 10.1074/jbc.M004175200.
72. Capell A, Steiner H, Willem M, et al. Maturation and pro-peptide cleavage of beta-secretase. *J Biol Chem* 2000;275:30849-54. DOI: 10.1074/jbc.M003202200.
73. Refolo LM, Malester B, LaFrancois J, et al. Hypercholesterolemia accelerates the Alzheimer's amyloid pathology in a transgenic mouse model. *Neurobiol Dis* 2000;7:321-31. DOI: 10.1006/nbdi.2000.0304.
74. Hartmann T, Kuchenbecker J, Grimm MO. Alzheimer's Disease: the lipid connection. *J Neurochem* 2007;103 Suppl 1:159-70. DOI: 10.1111/j.1471-4159.2007.04715.x.
75. Cao X, Sudhof TC. A transcriptionally [correction of transcriptively] active complex of APP with Fe65 and histone acetyltransferase Tip60. *Science* 2001;293:115-20. DOI: 10.1126/science.1058783.
76. Cupers P, Bentahir M, Craessaerts K, et al. The discrepancy between presenilin subcellular localization and gamma-secretase processing of amyloid precursor protein. *J Cell Biol* 2001;154:731-40. DOI: 10.1083/jcb.200104045.
77. Kimberly WT, Zheng JB, Guenette SY, Selkoe DJ. The intracellular domain of the beta-amyloid precursor protein is stabilized by Fe65 and translocates to the nucleus in a notch-like manner. *J Biol Chem* 2001;276:40288-92.
78. Yu G, Nishimura M, Arawaka S, et al. Nicastrin modulates presenilin-mediated notch/glp-1 signal transduction and betaAPP processing. *Nature* 2000;407:48-54. DOI: 10.1038/35024009.

79. Gu Y, Misonou H, Sato T, Dohmae N, Takio K, Ihara Y. Distinct intramembrane cleavage of the beta-amyloid precursor protein family resembling gamma-secretase-like cleavage of Notch. *J Biol Chem* 2001;276:35235-8. DOI: 10.1074/jbc.C100357200.
80. Sastre M, Steiner H, Fuchs K, et al. Presenilin-dependent gamma-secretase processing of beta-amyloid precursor protein at a site corresponding to the S3 cleavage of Notch. *EMBO Rep* 2001;2:835-41. DOI: 10.1093/embo-reports/kve180.
81. Kinoshita A, Whelan CM, Berezovska O, Hyman BT. The gamma secretase-generated carboxyl-terminal domain of the amyloid precursor protein induces apoptosis via Tip60 in H4 cells. *J Biol Chem* 2002;277:28530-6. DOI: 10.1074/jbc.M203372200.
82. Weidemann A, Eggert S, Reinhard FB, et al. A novel epsilon-cleavage within the transmembrane domain of the Alzheimer amyloid precursor protein demonstrates homology with Notch processing. *Biochemistry* 2002;41:2825-35. DOI: 10.1021/bi015794o.
83. Cao X, Sudhof TC. Dissection of amyloid-beta precursor protein-dependent transcriptional transactivation. *J Biol Chem* 2004;279:24601-11. DOI: 10.1074/jbc.M402248200.
84. De Strooper B, Saftig P, Craessaerts K, et al. Deficiency of presenilin-1 inhibits the normal cleavage of amyloid precursor protein. *Nature* 1998;391:387-90. DOI: 10.1038/34910.
85. Annaert WG, Levesque L, Craessaerts K, et al. Presenilin 1 controls gamma-secretase processing of amyloid precursor protein in pre-golgi compartments of hippocampal neurons. *J Cell Biol* 1999;147:277-94. DOI: 10.1083/jcb.147.2.277.
86. Haass C, Koo EH, Mellon A, Hung AY, Selkoe DJ. Targeting of cell-surface beta-amyloid precursor protein to lysosomes: alternative processing into amyloid-bearing fragments. *Nature* 1992;357:500-3. DOI: 10.1038/357500a0.
87. Higaki J, Quon D, Zhong Z, Cordell B. Inhibition of beta-amyloid formation identifies proteolytic precursors and subcellular site of catabolism. *Neuron* 1995;14:651-9. DOI: 10.1016/0896-6273(95)90322-4.
88. Cook DG, Forman MS, Sung JC, et al. Alzheimer's A beta(1-42) is generated in the endoplasmic reticulum/intermediate compartment of NT2N cells. *Nat Med* 1997;3:1021-3. DOI: 10.1038/nm0997-1021.
89. Hartmann T, Bieger SC, Bruhl B, et al. Distinct sites of intracellular production for Alzheimer's Disease A beta40/42 amyloid peptides. *Nat Med* 1997;3:1016-20. DOI: 10.1038/nm0997-1016.
90. Wild-Bode C, Yamazaki T, Capell A, et al. Intracellular generation and accumulation of amyloid beta-peptide terminating at amino acid 42. *J Biol Chem* 1997;272:16085-8. DOI: 10.1074/jbc.272.26.16085.

91. Perez RG, Soriano S, Hayes JD, et al. Mutagenesis identifies new signals for beta-amyloid precursor protein endocytosis, turnover, and the generation of secreted fragments, including Abeta42. *J Biol Chem* 1999;274:18851-6. DOI: 10.1074/jbc.274.27.18851.
92. Petit A, Bihel F, Alves da Costa C, Pourquie O, Checler F, Kraus JL. New protease inhibitors prevent gamma-secretase-mediated production of Abeta40/42 without affecting Notch cleavage. *Nat Cell Biol* 2001;3:507-11. DOI: 10.1038/35074581.
93. Dovey HF, Suomensaari-Chrysler S, Lieberburg I, Sinha S, Keim PS. Cells with a familial Alzheimer's Disease mutation produce authentic beta-peptide. *Neuroreport* 1993;4:1039-42. DOI: 10.1097/00001756-199308000-00011.
94. Wang R, Sweeney D, Gandy SE, Sisodia SS. The profile of soluble amyloid beta protein in cultured cell media. Detection and quantification of amyloid beta protein and variants by immunoprecipitation-mass spectrometry. *J Biol Chem* 1996;271:31894-902. DOI: 10.1074/jbc.271.50.31894.
95. Baumann K, Paganetti PA, Sturchler-Pierrat C, et al. Distinct processing of endogenous and overexpressed recombinant presenilin 1. *Neurobiol Aging* 1997;18:181-9. DOI: 10.1016/S0197-4580(97)00004-3.
96. De Strooper B, Beullens M, Contreras B, et al. Phosphorylation, subcellular localization, and membrane orientation of the Alzheimer's Disease-associated presenilins. *J Biol Chem* 1997;272:3590-8. DOI: 10.1074/jbc.272.6.3590.
97. Brunkan AL, Goate AM. Presenilin function and gamma-secretase activity. *J Neurochem* 2005;93:769-92. DOI: 10.1111/j.1471-4159.2005.03099.x.
98. Steiner H, Fluhrer R, Haass C. Intramembrane proteolysis by gamma-secretase. *J Biol Chem* 2008;283:29627-31. DOI: 10.1074/jbc.R800010200.
99. Vito P, Ghayur T, D'Adamio L. Generation of anti-apoptotic presenilin-2 polypeptides by alternative transcription, proteolysis, and caspase-3 cleavage. *J Biol Chem* 1997;272:28315-20. DOI: 10.1074/jbc.272.45.28315.
100. Wolozin B, Iwasaki K, Vito P, et al. Participation of presenilin 2 in apoptosis: enhanced basal activity conferred by an Alzheimer mutation. *Science* 1996;274:1710-3. DOI: 10.1126/science.274.5293.1710.
101. Kim TW, Pettingell WH, Jung YK, Kovacs DM, Tanzi RE. Alternative cleavage of Alzheimer-associated presenilins during apoptosis by a caspase-3 family protease. *Science* 1997;277:373-6. DOI: 10.1126/science.277.5324.373.
102. Walter J, Schindzielorz A, Grunberg J, Haass C. Phosphorylation of presenilin-2 regulates its cleavage by caspases and retards progression of apoptosis. *Proc Natl Acad Sci U S A* 1999;96:1391-6. DOI: 10.1073/pnas.96.4.1391.

103. Kimberly WT, Wolfe MS. Identity and function of gamma-secretase. *J Neurosci* Res 2003;74:353-60. DOI: 10.1002/jnr.10736.

104. Fortini ME. Gamma-secretase-mediated proteolysis in cell-surface-receptor signalling. *Nat Rev Mol Cell Biol* 2002;3:673-84. DOI: 10.1038/nrm910.

105. Sisodia SS, St George-Hyslop PH. gamma-Secretase, Notch, Abeta and Alzheimer's Disease: where do the presenilins fit in? *Nat Rev Neurosci* 2002;3:281-90. DOI: 10.1038/nrn785.

106. Postina R. Activation of alpha-secretase cleavage. *J Neurochem* 2012;120 Suppl 1:46-54. DOI: 10.1111/j.1471-4159.2011.07459.x.

107. Lannfelt L, Basun H, Wahlund LO, Rowe BA, Wagner SL. Decreased alpha-secretase-cleaved amyloid precursor protein as a diagnostic marker for Alzheimer's Disease. *Nat Med* 1995;1:829-32. DOI: 10.1038/nm0895-829.

108. Sennvik K, Fastbom J, Blomberg M, Wahlund LO, Winblad B, Benedikz E. Levels of alpha- and beta-secretase cleaved amyloid precursor protein in the cerebrospinal fluid of Alzheimer's Disease patients. *Neurosci Lett* 2000;278:169-72. DOI: 10.1016/S0304-3940(99)00929-5.

109. Esch FS, Keim PS, Beattie EC, et al. Cleavage of amyloid beta peptide during constitutive processing of its precursor. *Science* 1990;248:1122-4. DOI: 10.1126/science.2111583.

110. Sisodia SS, Koo EH, Beyreuther K, Unterbeck A, Price DL. Evidence that beta-amyloid protein in Alzheimer's Disease is not derived by normal processing. *Science* 1990;248:492-5. DOI: 10.1126/science.1691865.

111. Wang R, Meschia JF, Cotter RJ, Sisodia SS. Secretion of the beta/A4 amyloid precursor protein. Identification of a cleavage site in cultured mammalian cells. *J Biol Chem* 1991;266:16960-4.

112. Streltsov VA, Varghese JN, Masters CL, Nuttall SD. Crystal structure of the amyloid-beta p3 fragment provides a model for oligomer formation in Alzheimer's Disease. *J Neurosci* 2011;31:1419-26. DOI: 10.1523/JNEUROSCI.4259-10.2011.

113. Jang H, Arce FT, Ramachandran S, et al. Truncated beta-amyloid peptide channels provide an alternative mechanism for Alzheimer's Disease and Down syndrome. *Proc Natl Acad Sci U S A* 2010;107:6538-43. DOI: 10.1073/pnas.0914251107.

114. Kumar-Singh S, Theuns J, Van Broeck B, et al. Mean age-of-onset of familial Alzheimer's Disease caused by presenilin mutations correlates with both increased Abeta42 and decreased Abeta40. Hum Mutat 2006;27:686-95. DOI: 10.1002/humu.20336.

115. Bentahir M, Nyabi O, Verhamme J, et al. Presenilin clinical mutations can affect gamma-secretase activity by different mechanisms. *J Neurochem* 2006;96:732-42. DOI: 10.1111/j.1471-4159.2005.03578.x.

116. Jonsson T, Atwal JK, Steinberg S, et al. A mutation in APP protects against Alzheimer's Disease and age-related cognitive decline. *Nature* 2012;488:96-9. DOI: 10.1038/nature11283.

117. Zhu X, Lee HG, Moreira PI, Smith MA, Perry G. Presenilin mutation: a deadly first hit in Alzheimer's Disease. A commentary on "aging sensitizes towards ROS formation and lipid peroxidation in PS1M146L transgenic mice." *Free Radic Biol Med* 2006;40:737-9. DOI: 10.1016/j.freeradbiomed.2005.12.028.

118. Haass C, Lemere CA, Capell A, et al. The Swedish mutation causes early-onset Alzheimer's Disease by beta-secretase cleavage within the secretory pathway. *Nat Med* 1995;1:1291-6. DOI: 10.1038/nm1295-1291.

119. Larner AJ, Doran M. Clinical phenotypic heterogeneity of Alzheimer's Disease associated with mutations of the presenilin-1 gene. *J Neurol* 2006;253:139-58. DOI: 10.1007/s00415-005-0019-5.

120. Mendez MF, McMurtray A. Frontotemporal dementia-like phenotypes associated with presenilin-1 mutations. *Am J Alzheimers Dis Other Demen* 2006;21:281-6. DOI: 10.1177/1533317506290448.

121. Riudavets MA, Bartoloni L, Troncoso JC, et al. Familial Dementia With Frontotemporal Features Associated With M146V Presenilin-1 Mutation. *Brain Pathol* 2013;23:595-600. DOI: 10.1111/bpa.12051.

122. Verkkoniemi A, Kalimo H, Paetau A, et al. Variant Alzheimer's Disease with spastic paraparesis: neuropathological phenotype. *J Neuropathol Exp Neurol* 2001;60:483-92.

123. Lemere CA, Lopera F, Kosik KS, et al. The E280A presenilin 1 Alzheimer mutation produces increased A beta 42 deposition and severe cerebellar pathology. *Nat Med* 1996;2:1146-50. DOI: 10.1038/nm1096-1146.

124. Levy E, Carman MD, Fernandez-Madrid IJ, et al. Mutation of the Alzheimer's Disease amyloid gene in hereditary cerebral hemorrhage, Dutch type. *Science* 1990;248:1124-6. DOI: 10.1126/science.2111584.

125. Snider BJ, Norton J, Coats MA, et al. Novel presenilin 1 mutation (S170F) causing Alzheimer's Disease with Lewy bodies in the third decade of life. *Arch Neurol* 2005;62:1821-30. DOI: 10.1001/archneur.62.12.1821.

126. Cras P, van Harskamp F, Hendriks L, et al. Presenile Alzheimer's Dementia characterized by amyloid angiopathy and large amyloid core type senile plaques in the APP 692Ala-->Gly mutation. *Acta Neuropathol* 1998;96:253-60. DOI: 10.1007/s004010050892.

127. Verghese PB, Castellano JM, Holtzman DM. Apolipoprotein E in Alzheimer's Disease and other neurological disorders. *Lancet Neurol* 2011;10:241-52. DOI: 10.1016/S1474-4422(10)70325-2.

128. Berg L, McKeel DW, Jr., Miller JP, et al. Clinicopathologic studies in cognitively healthy aging and Alzheimer's Disease: relation of histologic markers to dementia severity, age, sex, and apolipoprotein E genotype. *Arch Neurol* 1998;55:326-35. DOI: 10.1001/archneur.55.3.326.

129. Vidal R, Calero M, Piccardo P, et al. Senile dementia associated with amyloid beta protein angiopathy and tau perivascular pathology but not neuritic plaques in patients homozygous for the APOE-epsilon4 allele. *Acta Neuropathol* 2000;100:1-12. DOI: 10.1007/s004010051186.

130. Braak H, Thal DR, Ghebremedhin E, Del Tredici K. Stages of the pathologic process in Alzheimer's Disease: age categories from 1 to 100 years. *J Neuropathol Exp Neurol* 2011;70:960-9. DOI: 10.1097/NEN.0b013e318232a379.

131. McKee AC, Stein TD, Nowinski CJ, et al. The spectrum of disease in chronic traumatic encephalopathy. *Brain* 2013;136:43-64.

132. Spires-Jones TL, Stoothoff WH, de Calignon A, Jones PB, Hyman BT. Tau pathophysiology in neurodegeneration: a tangled issue. *Trends Neurosci* 2009;32:150-9. DOI: 10.1016/j.tins.2008.11.007.

133. Castellani RJ, Nunomura A, Lee HG, Perry G, Smith MA. Phosphorylated tau: toxic, protective, or none of the above. *J Alzheimers Dis* 2008;14:377-83.

134. Divry P. J Belge *Neurol et Psychiat* 1934;134:726.

135. Kidd M. Paired helical filaments in electron microscopy of Alzheimer's Disease. *Nature* 1963;197:192-3. DOI: 10.1038/197192b0.

136. Iqbal K, Zaidi T, Thompson CH, Merz PA, Wisniewski HM. Alzheimer paired helical filaments: bulk isolation, solubility, and protein composition. *Acta Neuropathol* 1984;62:167-77. DOI: 10.1007/BF00691849.

137. Grundke-Iqbal I, Iqbal K, Tung YC, Wisniewski HM. Alzheimer paired helical filaments: immunochemical identification of polypeptides. *Acta Neuropathol* 1984;62:259-67. DOI: 10.1007/BF00687607.

138. Grundke-Iqbal I, Iqbal K, Quinlan M, Tung YC, Zaidi MS, Wisniewski HM. Microtubule-associated protein tau. A component of Alzheimer paired helical filaments. *J Biol Chem* 1986;261:6084-9.

139. Grundke-Iqbal I, Iqbal K, Tung YC, Quinlan M, Wisniewski HM, Binder LI. Abnormal phosphorylation of the microtubule-associated protein tau (tau) in Alzheimer cytoskeletal pathology. *Proc Natl Acad Sci U S A* 1986;83:4913-7. DOI: 10.1073/pnas.83.13.4913.

140. Kolarova M, Garcia-Sierra F, Bartos A, Ricny J, Ripova D. Structure and pathology of tau protein in Alzheimer's Disease. Int *J Alzheimers Dis* 2012;2012:731526. DOI: 10.1155/2012/731526.

141. Wolfe MS. Tau mutations in neurodegenerative diseases. *J Biol Chem* 2009;284:6021-5. DOI: 10.1074/jbc.R800013200.

142. Mulvihill P, Perry G. Immunoaffinity demonstration that paired helical filaments of Alzheimer's Disease share epitopes with neurofilaments, MAP2 and tau. *Brain Res* 1989;484:150-6. DOI: 10.1016/0006-8993(89)90357-0.

143. Voss K, Gamblin TC. GSK-3beta phosphorylation of functionally distinct tau isoforms has differential, but mild effects. *Mol Neurodegener* 2009;4:18. DOI: 10.1186/1750-1326-4-18.

144. Simchowicz T. Histologische Studien uber die senile Demenz. *Histologische and histopathologische Arbeiten uber die Grosshirnrinde* 1911;4:267-444.

145. Tomlinson BE, Kitchener D. Granulovacuolar degeneration of hippocampal pyramidal cells. *J Pathol* 1972;106:165-85. DOI: 10.1002/path.1711060305.

146. Hirano A, Malamud N, Elizan TS, Kurland LT. Amyotrophic lateral sclerosis and Parkinsonism-dementia complex on Guam. Further pathologic studies. *Arch Neurol* 1966;15:35-51. DOI: 10.1001/archneur.1966.00470130039004.

147. Hirano A, Tuazon R, Zimmerman HM. Neurofibrillary changes, granulovacuolar bodies and argentophilic globules observed in tuberous sclerosis. *Acta Neuropathol* 1968;11:257-61.

148. Ball MJ, Vis CL. Relationship of granulovacuolar degeneration in hippocampal neurones to aging and to dementia in normal-pressure hydrocephalics. *J Gerontol* 1978;33:815-24. DOI: 10.1093/geronj/33.6.815.

149. Esiri MM, Wilcock GK. The olfactory bulbs in Alzheimer's Disease. *J Neurol* Neurosurg Psychiatry 1984;47:56-60. DOI: 10.1136/jnnp.47.1.56.

150. Anderton BH, Breinburg D, Downes MJ, et al. Monoclonal antibodies show that neurofibrillary tangles and neurofilaments share antigenic determinants. *Nature* 1982;298:84-6. DOI: 10.1038/298084a0.

151. Mann DM. Granulovacuolar degeneration in pyramidal cells of the hippocampus. *Acta Neuropathol* 1978;42:149-51. DOI: 10.1007/BF00690983.

152. Vincent I, Zheng JH, Dickson DW, Kress Y, Davies P. Mitotic phosphoepitopes precede paired helical filaments in Alzheimer's Disease. *Neurobiol Aging* 1998;19:287-96. DOI: 10.1016/S0197-4580(98)00071-2.

153. Lagalwar S, Berry RW, Binder LI. Relation of hippocampal phospho-SAPK/JNK granules in Alzheimer's Disease and tauopathies to granulovacuolar degeneration bodies. *Acta Neuropathol* 2007;113:63-73. DOI: 10.1007/s00401-006-0159-4.

154. Dakson A, Yokota O, Esiri M, et al. Granular expression of prolyl-peptidyl isomerase PIN1 is a constant and specific feature of Alzheimer's Disease pathology and is independent of tau, Abeta and TDP-43 pathology. *Acta Neuropathol* 2011;121:635-49. DOI: 10.1007/s00401-011-0798-y.

155. Perry G, Roder H, Nunomura A, et al. Activation of neuronal extracellular receptor kinase (ERK) in Alzheimer's Disease links oxidative stress to abnormal phosphorylation. *Neuroreport* 1999;10:2411-5. DOI: 10.1097/00001756-199908020-00035.

156. Yamazaki Y, Takahashi T, Hiji M, et al. Immunopositivity for ESCRT-III subunit CHMP2B in granulovacuolar degeneration of neurons in the Alzheimer's Disease hippocampus. *Neurosci Lett* 2010;477:86-90. DOI: 10.1016/j.neulet.2010.04.038.

157. Funk KE, Mrak RE, Kuret J. Granulovacuolar degeneration (GVD) bodies of Alzheimer's Disease (AD) resemble late-stage autophagic organelles. *Neuropathol Appl Neurobiol* 2011;37:295-306. DOI: 10.1111/j.1365-2990.2010.01135.x.

158. Hoozemans JJ, van Haastert ES, Nijholt DA, Rozemuller AJ, Eikelenboom P, Scheper W. The unfolded protein response is activated in pretangle neurons in Alzheimer's Disease hippocampus. Am *J Pathol* 2009;174:1241-51. DOI: 10.2353/ajpath.2009.080814.

159. Ball MJ. Neuronal loss, neurofibrillary tangles and granulovacuolar degeneration in the hippocampus with ageing and dementia. A quantitative study. *Acta Neuropathol* 1977;37:111-8. DOI: 10.1007/BF00692056.

160. Holzer M, Gartner U, Stobe A, et al. Inverse association of Pin1 and tau accumulation in Alzheimer's Disease hippocampus. *Acta Neuropathol* 2002;104:471-81.

161. Castellani RJ, Gupta Y, Sheng B, et al. A novel origin for granulovacuolar degeneration in aging and Alzheimer's Disease: parallels to stress granules. *Lab Invest* 2011;91:1777-86. DOI: 10.1038/labinvest.2011.149.

162. Anderson P, Kedersha N. Stress granules. *Curr Biol* 2009;19:R397-8. DOI: 10.1016/j.cub.2009.03.013.

163. Cande C, Vahsen N, Metivier D, et al. Regulation of cytoplasmic stress granules by apoptosis-inducing factor. *J Cell Sci* 2004;117:4461-8. DOI: 10.1242/jcs.01356.

164. Braak H, Braak E. Neuropathological stageing of Alzheimer-related changes. *Acta Neuropathol* 1991;82:239-59. DOI: 10.1007/BF00308809.

165. Schonheit B, Zarski R, Ohm TG. Spatial and temporal relationships between plaques and tangles in Alzheimer-pathology. *Neurobiol Aging* 2004;25:697-711. DOI: 10.1016/j.neurobiolaging.2003.09.009.

166. Teller JK, Russo C, DeBusk LM, et al. Presence of soluble amyloid beta-peptide precedes amyloid plaque formation in Down's syndrome. *Nat Med* 1996;2:93-5. DOI: 10.1038/nm0196-93.

167. Berg L, McKeel DW, Jr., Miller JP, Baty J, Morris JC. Neuropathological indexes of Alzheimer's Disease in demented and nondemented persons aged 80 years and older. *Arch Neurol* 1993;50:349-58. DOI: 10.1001/archneur.1993.00540040011008.

168. Giannakopoulos P, Herrmann FR, Bussiere T, et al. Tangle and neuron numbers, but not amyloid load, predict cognitive status in Alzheimer's Disease. *Neurology* 2003;60:1495-500. DOI: 10.1212/01.WNL.0000063311.58879.01.

169. Knopman DS, Parisi JE, Salviati A, et al. Neuropathology of cognitively normal elderly. *J Neuropathol Exp Neurol* 2003;62:1087-95.

170. Redlich E. Uber miliare Sklerose der Hirnrinde bei seniler Atrophie. *Psychiat Neurol* 1898;17:208-16.

171. Walsh DM, Selkoe DJ. A beta oligomers - a decade of discovery. *J Neurochem* 2007;101:1172-84. DOI: 10.1111/j.1471-4159.2006.04426.x.

172. Benilova I, Karran E, De Strooper B. The toxic Abeta oligomer and Alzheimer's Disease: an emperor in need of clothes. *Nat Neurosci* 2012;15:349-57. DOI: 10.1038/nn.3028.

173. Stephan BC, Hunter S, Harris D, et al. The neuropathological profile of mild cognitive impairment (MCI): a systematic review. *Mol Psychiatry* 2011;17:1056-76. DOI: 10.1038/mp.2011.147.

174. Castellani RJ, Rolston RK, Smith MA. Alzheimer's Disease. *Dis Mon* 2010;56:484-546. DOI: 10.1016/j.disamonth.2010.06.001.

175. Terry RD, Masliah E, Salmon DP, et al. Physical basis of cognitive alterations in Alzheimer's Disease: synapse loss is the major correlate of cognitive impairment. *Ann Neurol* 1991;30:572-80. DOI: 10.1002/ana.410300410.

176. Nordberg A. Amyloid plaque imaging in vivo: current achievement and future prospects. *Eur J Nucl Med Mol Imaging* 2008;35 Suppl 1:S46-50. DOI: 10.1007/s00259-007-0700-2.

177. Balasubramanian AB, Kawas CH, Peltz CB, Brookmeyer R, Corrada MM. Alzheimer's Disease pathology and longitudinal cognitive performance in the oldest-old with no dementia. *Neurology*;79:915-21. DOI: 10.1212/WNL.0b013e318266fc77.

178. Braak H, Thal DR, Ghebremedhin E, Del Tredici K. Stages of the pathologic process in Alzheimer's Disease: age categories from 1 to 100 years. *J Neuropathol Exp Neurol*;70:960-9. DOI: 10.1097/NEN.0b013e318232a379.

179. Nelson PT, Alafuzoff I, Bigio EH, et al. Correlation of Alzheimer's Disease neuropathologic changes with cognitive status: a review of the literature. *J Neuropathol Exp Neurol*;71:362-81. DOI: 10.1097/NEN.0b013e31825018f7.

180. Arnold SE, Hyman BT, Flory J, Damasio AR, Van Hoesen GW. The topographical and neuroanatomical distribution of neurofibrillary tangles and neuritic plaques in the cerebral cortex of patients with Alzheimer's Disease. *Cereb Cortex* 1991;1:103-16. DOI: 10.1093/cercor/1.1.103.

181. Dickson DW, Crystal HA, Mattiace LA, et al. Identification of normal and pathological aging in prospectively studied nondemented elderly humans. *Neurobiol Aging* 1992;13:179-89. DOI: 10.1016/0197-4580(92)90027-U.

182. Haroutunian V, Purohit DP, Perl DP, et al. Neurofibrillary tangles in nondemented elderly subjects and mild Alzheimer's Disease. *Arch Neurol* 1999;56:713-8. DOI: 10.1001/archneur.56.6.713.

183. Blessed G, Tomlinson BE, Roth M. The association between quantitative measures of dementia and of senile change in the cerebral grey matter of elderly subjects. *Br J Psychiatry* 1968;114:797-811. DOI: 10.1192/bjp.114.512.797.

184. Glatt SL, Hubble JP, Lyons K, et al. Risk factors for dementia in Parkinson's disease: effect of education. *Neuroepidemiology* 1996;15:20-5. DOI: 10.1159/000109885.

185. Beard CM, Kokmen E, Offord KP, Kurland LT. Lack of association between Alzheimer's Disease and education, occupation, marital status, or living arrangement. *Neurology* 1992;42:2063-8. DOI: 10.1212/WNL.42.11.2063.

186. Cobb JL, Wolf PA, Au R, White R, D'Agostino RB. The effect of education on the incidence of dementia and Alzheimer's Disease in the Framingham Study. *Neurology* 1995;45:1707-12. DOI: 10.1212/WNL.45.9.1707.

187. Farias ST, Chand V, Bonnici L, et al. Idea density measured in late life predicts subsequent cognitive trajectories: implications for the measurement of cognitive reserve. *J Gerontol B Psychol Sci Soc Sci* 2012;67:677-86. DOI: 10.1093/geronb/gbr162.

188. Riley KP, Snowdon DA, Desrosiers MF, Markesbery WR. Early life linguistic ability, late life cognitive function, and neuropathology: findings from the Nun Study. *Neurobiol Aging* 2005;26:341-7. DOI: 10.1016/j.neurobiolaging.2004.06.019.

189. Stein PS, Desrosiers M, Donegan SJ, Yepes JF, Kryscio RJ. Tooth loss, dementia and neuropathology in the Nun study. *J Am Dent Assoc* 2007;138:1314-22; quiz 81-2.

190. Bickel H, Kurz A. Education, occupation, and dementia: the Bavarian school sisters study. *Dement Geriatr Cogn Disord* 2009;27:548-56. DOI: 10.1159/000227781.

191. Khachaturian ZS. Diagnosis of Alzheimer's Disease. *Arch Neurol* 1985;42:1097-105. DOI: 10.1001/archneur.1985.04060100083029.

192. Hyman BT, Trojanowski JQ. Consensus recommendations for the postmortem diagnosis of Alzheimer's Disease from the National Institute on Aging and the Reagan Institute Working Group on diagnostic criteria for the neuropathological assessment of Alzheimer's Disease. *J Neuropathol Exp Neurol* 1997;56:1095-7. DOI: 10.1097/00005072-199710000-00002.

193. Montine TJ, Phelps CH, Beach TG, et al. National Institute on Aging-Alzheimer's Association guidelines for the neuropathologic assessment of Alzheimer's Disease: a practical approach. *Acta Neuropathol* 2012;123:1-11. DOI: 10.1007/s00401-011-0910-3.

194. Thal DR, Rub U, Orantes M, Braak H. Phases of A beta-deposition in the human brain and its relevance for the development of AD. *Neurology* 2002;58:1791-800. DOI: 10.1212/WNL.58.12.1791.

195. Nelson PT, Braak H, Markesbery WR. Neuropathology and cognitive impairment in Alzheimer's Disease: a complex but coherent relationship. *J Neuropathol Exp Neurol* 2009;68:1-14. DOI: 10.1097/NEN.0b013e3181919a48.

196. Castellani RJ, Moreira PI, Perry G, Zhu X. The role of iron as a mediator of oxidative stress in Alzheimer's Disease. *Biofactors* 2012;38:133-8. DOI: 10.1002/biof.1010.

197. Jensen ON. Modification-specific proteomics: characterization of post-translational modifications by mass spectrometry. *Curr Opin Chem Biol* 2004;8:33-41. DOI: 10.1016/j.cbpa.2003.12.009.

198. Smith MA, Atwood CS, Joseph JA, Perry G. Ill-fated amyloid-beta vaccine. *J Neurosci Res* 2002;69:285. DOI: 10.1002/jnr.10316.

199. Graeber MB, Mehraein P. Reanalysis of the first case of Alzheimer's Disease. *Eur Arch Psychiatry Clin Neurosci* 1999;249 Suppl 3:10-3. DOI: 10.1007/PL00014167.

200. Berrios GE. Presbyophrenia: the rise and fall of a concept. *Psychol Med* 1986;16:267-75. DOI: 10.1017/S0033291700009089.

201. Castellani RJ, Smith MA, Perry G, Friedland RP. Cerebral amyloid angiopathy: major contributor or decorative response to Alzheimer's Disease pathogenesis. *Neurobiol Aging* 2004;25:599-602; discussion 3-4. DOI: 10.1016/j.neurobiolaging.2003.12.019.

202. Spillantini MG, Goedert M. Tau pathology and neurodegeneration. *Lancet Neurol* 2013;12:609-22. DOI: 10.1016/S1474-4422(13)70090-5.

203. Jucker M, Walker LC. Pathogenic protein seeding in Alzheimer's Disease and other neurodegenerative disorders. *Ann Neurol* 2011;70:532-40. DOI: 10.1002/ana.22615.

204. Montine TJ, Phelps CH, Beach TG, et al. National Institute on Aging-Alzheimer's Association guidelines for the neuropathologic assessment of Alzheimer's Disease: a practical approach. *Acta Neuropathol*;123:1-11. DOI: 10.1007/s00401-011-0910-3.

Author Biographies

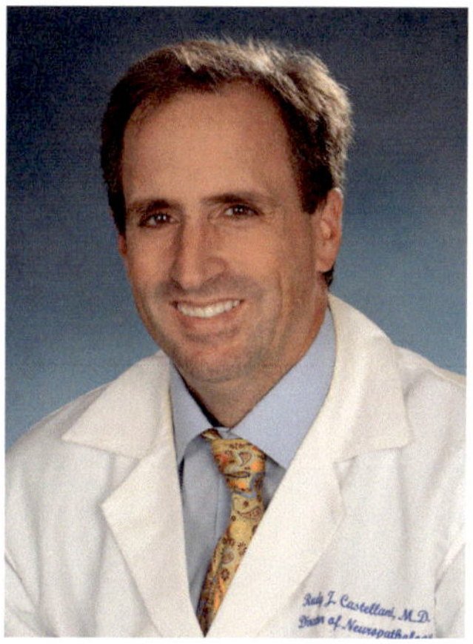

Dr. Rudolph J. Castellani is tenured professor of pathology and director of neuropathology at the University of Maryland School of Medicine. Dr. Castellani is the recipient of numerous awards for scientific merit, clinical service, and teaching, including the 2010 Alzheimer Medal, the 2011 Harlan I. Firminger award for excellence in pathology teaching, and Castle Connolly Medical Ltd. recognition as regional Top Doctor, 2013. His main fields of interest include neuropathology and pathogenesis of neurodegenerative diseases, prion diseases, and neurotrauma. He has published over 200 peer-reviewed papers, chapters, reviews, and books.

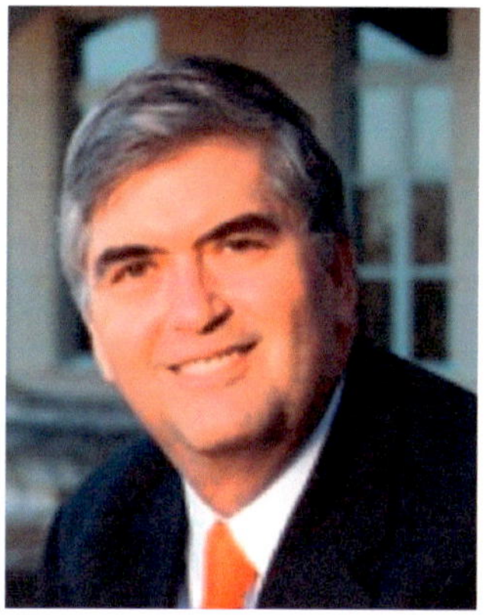

George Perry, Ph.D., is Dean of the College of Sciences and Professor of Biology at the University of Texas at San Antonio. He obtained his Ph.D. from Scripps Institution of Oceanography in 1979 and received a postdoctoral fellowship in the Department of Cell Biology at Baylor College of Medicine where he laid the foundation for his observations of abnormalities in cell structures. Dr. Perry is distinguished as one of the top Alzheimer's Disease researchers with over 1,000 publications, one of the top 100 most-cited scientists in neuroscience and behavior, and one of the top 25 scientists in free radical research. He is editor for numerous journals and is editor-in-chief for the *Journal of Alzheimer's Disease*. Internationally recognized, he is a Foreign Correspondent Member of the Spanish Royal Academy of Sciences, the Academy of Science Lisbon, and a Foreign Member of the Mexican National Academy of Sciences. He is also a recent recipient of the National Plaque of Honor from the Republic of Panama Ministry of Science and Technology. Dr. Perry's research is primarily focused on how Alzheimer's Disease develops and the physiological consequences of the disease at a cellular level. He is currently working to determine the sequence of events leading to damage caused by and the source of increased oxygen radicals along with routes to provide more effective treatment.

Made in the USA
Monee, IL
12 September 2026

62976958R00057